Paleo on the Cheap

Saving Time and Money
While Saving Your Health

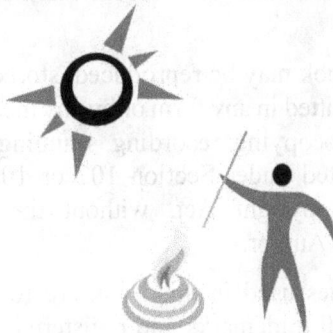

Harmony
Clearwater Grace

Paleo on the Cheap

Dear Friends,

Some of you may be surprised that I have written a book on a subject other than HCG. Don't be. I have great enthusiasm for all things that can optimize health, with the Paleo or Primal or Ancestral style of eating being just one of those things.

The concern that I hear so often from folks when I recommend eating Paleo or Primal, is that they don't think that they can afford it. They think that they must eat organic vegetables and fruit or that they must eat pastured butter and cage-free eggs, or only eat grass-fed meat. Optimally, of course, you would eat those things because they are unquestionably better quality.

But what if you are on a tight budget? What if even giving up one of your family cars wouldn't make it possible to buy your whole family those foods? Do you just give up and eat the Standard American Diet of grains, refined or processed foods, and junk food our bodies were never designed to eat?

I don't think so. That's why I decided to write this book, spurred on by questions from readers who didn't think that they could eat ancestrally, because they felt that they just couldn't afford it. In fact, the Paleo that you CAN or WILL do is going to make a difference in your health, versus the Perfect Paleo that won't happen AT ALL for you. As Voltaire said, "The perfect is the enemy of the good." Eating as Paleo as you can manage is still better than most Americans' diets.

Blessings with Love,

Harmony

P. S. Always remember: You DESERVE to be thin and healthy!

3

About the Author

In her newest book, *Paleo on the Cheap*, Harmony Clearwater Grace solves the problem of how to follow the Paleo or Primal Diet in order to be healthy without breaking your budget. Harmony is also the author of the bestselling books <u>HCG Diet Made Simple</u> and <u>The HCG Diet Book of Secrets</u>.

Harmony's vision is to be a catalyst to a complete turnaround of the current obesity epidemic and health crisis through her work.

Photo Attributions:

Table of Contents

Acknowledgements

Thank you to my true friends who lift me up and never bring me down, without whom this book would not be a reality.

Whenever possible, I cite references to support my opinions, either from the internet or clinical studies. When I cite references from the internet, I include a shortened URL using TinyURLs throughout this book for your convenience in using the URL links with minimum keystrokes. These URL references are not necessary for full understanding of my reasoning, but provide the actual research links that I used, in case you would like to read further background. As time goes on, the websites for those URLs may be changed or deleted altogether, as the internet is not a static reference, nor under my direct control in terms of how it changes. If you find that any URL link in this book no longer works, I apologize in advance, for these conditions beyond my control. If reported to me as a broken link, I will update the TinyURLs according to page number at this Web page:

http://www.paleoonthecheap.com/updates.html.

If you have any questions or concerns about the data in this book, I am always available through email to offer whatever help and support that I can. I am also very interested in hearing your story and how this information has helped you. Please be aware, however, that I am not a medical professional and that I cannot answer medical questions.

We only recommend products that we've either personally checked out ourselves or that come from people we know and trust. For doing so, we may receive compensation. Results are unique. Your results may vary.

.

Paleo on the Cheap

If you really want to eat Paleo style, but think that you just can't afford it, this book will help you to understand that anyone that can afford to EAT at all, can afford to eat PALEO.

You'll learn:

- The 10 rules of Paleo cost-effectiveness
- Practical ways to avoid paying retail
- The 7 best tricks for getting the best food cheaper
- How to expense-shift to save money to use for Paleo choices
- 3 secrets to making food last longer
- How to lower your expenses using social strategies and homemade helpers
- 7 sources for discounts and coupons
- Convenient formulas for freezing foods you might not have thought to freeze
- Learn which equipment purchases will save you money in the long run

Paleo Doesn't Have to Be Budget-Breaking

Chapter 1

You might have investigated the Paleo Diet and thought to yourself, "I'd have to be a millionaire to eat that way!" SURPRISE! You CAN eat Paleo style and still pay your mortgage or rent!

Many of you may know me from my books on the HCG Diet: *HCG Diet Made Simple* and *The HCG Diet Book of Secrets*. You might have even e-mailed me to ask questions about how to eat for your best health. I don't believe in a "one size fits all" type of diet that is best for everyone, but I do have certain ideas, based on years of research, about what foods should never be eaten by anyone, such as refined or highly processed types of foods and food additives such as MSG, HFCS, or artificial sweeteners. The Paleo or Primal diet certainly fits the bill to exclude those! If someone asks me for advice about how to eat for health, I don't hesitate to tell them to use Paleo as a starting place. Even vegetarians and vegans can eat somewhat Paleo style (with some extra effort), believe it or not!

How Did the Paleo/Primal/Ancestral Eating Movement Get Started?

Way back in 1975, Dr. Walter Veogtlin, a gastroenterologist, self-published a book he called *The Stone Age Diet*, in which he stated that the original human diet was carnivorous and included plenty of fat, due to it being animal-derived food. Then in 1985, Dr. S. Boyd Eaton wrote a paper entitled "Paleolithic Nutrition" published in the New England Journal of Medicine, explaining that our genetic programming should determine our optimal diet, since our DNA has changed little since Paleo times. The first book that I ever read about Paleo was by Ray Audette, and was called NeanderThin. Written in 1999, this book is now out of print, but can be bought used.

Ray built on the work of Dr. Eaton, saying that he ate only food that would be edible when raw AND was readily available in the Paleolithic age with only a sharp stick or stone.

More recently, the books of Dr. Loren Cordain, who was consulted for Ray's book, Robb Wolf, a research biochemist and conditioning coach, and Mark Sisson, a health and fitness expert, have brought Paleo to the masses. In fact, only 12% of those in a recent Paleo survey have been eating Paleo for more than two years, with 43% having learned about Paleo in 2010, as opposed to 26% in 2009 and 10% in 2008. Many of these folks first heard of Paleo or Primal eating through blogs.

Once people are convinced that Paleo is a healthy choice for them, they begin to notice that eating only organic fruits and vegetables, only grass-fed beef, wild fish, and organic free-range chickens, costs more than the other kinds of less healthy mainstream food that they had been buying before.

This book will help you learn HOW to affordably eat Paleo foods, WHAT is needed in order to find them most cheaply, WHICH foods can most safely be bought non-organically, and exactly WHERE to find the supplies you need to stretch your Paleo/Primal food dollar. In this book, it's all "done for you" so that you know what you can do to put Paleo into practice in your life less expensively. I've made it even simpler for you, by creating an online store for the more difficult to find items:

http://paleodieterstore.com/

Paleo Shopping List

One of the most difficult parts of writing this book is that Paleo is defined differently by different authors, so some folks are eating things that others would not eat to be strict Paleo. I'm perfectly fine with this because, as I wrote earlier, I don't think that one diet fits all. That also means that one Paleo Diet won't fit all, either. For instance, some eat dairy, others eat only raw dairy, some only certain kinds of dairy, while others eat no dairy at all. Some use artificial sweeteners, some use only honey and others use only natural sweeteners such as stevia. There are those such as Dr. Paul Jaminet that include potato or rice as "safe starches," others use only sweet potatoes or yams, and some eat none at all. Then there's Paleo 1.0, Paleo 1.5, Paleo 2.0, and finally, Paleo 3.0.

Paleo 1.0 could be thought of as the diet promoted by Audette, Cordain, Wolf, and Sisson, with no grains, no dairy (mostly), no sugar, no beans or legumes, no potatoes, and nothing else that could not or would not have been eaten by our Paleolithic ancestors. In Neaderthin, Ray Audette defined Paleo as eating what would be obtainable by using a sharp stick or a stone and edible in that state. No technology allowed. It should be noted that Sisson allows occasional non-Paleo indulgences, using the 80/20 rule.

Dr. Art DeVany has a variation that might be considered to be Paleo 1.5, in which he marries Mediterranean with Paleo.

Kurt Harris has formulated what could be called Paleo 2.0, which includes more foods and aims to avoid Neolithic agents of disease more than to emulate the exact diet of our ancestors. Just which foods are acceptable is a matter of contention, however, with some authors and bloggers allowing certain foods and others allowing others, with little agreement and lots of confusion. What they all have in common is a lack of refined and processed foods.

Dr. Jack Kruse and Robert Haas have developed ways of eating for compatibility with individual genes and gene switches, typically guided by blood test results designed to gauge how diet and lifestyle changes are affecting health markers that indicate epigenetic changes, both favorable and unfavorable. This personalized version is regarded as Paleo 3.0, although it is really more about eating for epigenetics.

Then there's ketogenic Paleo and Primal. Whew! Because I know that eating Paleo style is not a "One Paleo fits all" proposition, I'm going to be more inclusive rather than limiting in my list. Therefore, I want you to feel free to omit anything that you don't choose to eat as Paleo.

Meats

Beef, bison, goat, horse, lamb, pork, sheep, and veal

Game Meats

Alligator, bear, bison, caribou, deer, duck, elk, goat, goose, kangaroo, ostrich, moose, pheasant, quail, rattlesnake, reindeer, rabbit, reindeer, squab, turtle, venison, wild boar, wild turkey, and woodcock

Poultry

Chicken, duck, goose, quail, and turkey

Fish

Anchovy, bass, bluefish, carp, cod, drum, eel, flatfish, grouper, haddock, halibut, herring, mackerel, monkfish, mullet, pike, orange roughy, perch, red snapper, salmon, sardines, scrod, shark, sole, sunfish, tilapia, trout, tuna, turbot, walleye, and whitefish

Shellfish

Abalone, clam, crab, crawfish, lobster, mussel, octopus, oyster, scallop, shrimp, and squid.

Fats

Avocados, avocado oil, butter, clarified butter (ghee), coconut flesh, coconut oil, coconut milk, duck fat, fatty fishes (sardines, mackerel, salmon), heavy whipping cream, lamb fat, lard, nut butters, nut oils (walnut, macadamia),olives and olive oil, tallow, and veal fat

Eggs

Chicken eggs, duck eggs, goose eggs, and quail eggs

Vegetables

Artichokes, asparagus, avocados, beets, bell peppers, broccoli, Brussels sprouts, cabbage, cauliflower, celery, cucumber, eggplants, green beans (Robb Wolf signed off on this one in a podcast), green onions, nopales, kohlrabi, leeks, okra, onions, peppers, purslane, rhubarb, seaweed, tomatillos, and tomatoes

Green Leafy Vegetables

Arugula (rocket), bok choy, beet top, chicory, collard greens, dandelion, endive, kale, lettuce, mustard greens, radicchio, rapini, spinach, Swiss chard, turnip greens, and watercress

Root Vegetables

Beets, carrots, yucca (cassava), turnips, parsnips, radish, rutabaga, sweet potatoes, jerusalem artichokes, jicama, and yams

Winter Squash

Acorn squash, buttercup squash, butternut squash, pumpkin, and spaghetti squash

Summer Squash

Yellow, crookneck squash, and zucchini

Fruits

Apple, apricot, banana, berry (blackberry, blueberry, boysenberry, cranberry, gooseberry raspberry, strawberry), cantaloupe, cherimoya, cherry, currant, date, fig, grape, grapefruit, guava, kiwi, lemon, lime, lychee, mango, melon, nectarine, orange, papaya, passion fruit, peach, pear, persimmon, pineapple, plantain, plum, pomegranate, star fruit (carambola), tangelo, and tangerine

Nuts and Seeds

Acorn, almond, Brazil nut, caraway, cashew, celery, chervil, chestnut, coconut, cumin, fennel, filbert, flax, hazelnut, hickory, macadamia nut, mustard, pecan, pine nut, pistachio, poppy, pumpkin seed (pepita), sesame seed, sunflower seed, and walnut

Mushrooms

Button mushroom, chanterelle, crimini, morel, oyster mushroom, porcini, Portobello, and shiitake

Fresh and Dried Herbs

Basil, bay leaves, chives, coriander, dill, lavender, mint, oregano, parsley, rosemary, sage, tarragon, and thyme

Herbs and Spices and Other Natural Flavor Enhancers

Black pepper, cayenne pepper, chilies, cilantro, cinnamon, cloves, cumin, fennel seed, garlic, ginger, hot pepper, mustard seed, onion, nutmeg, paprika, parsley, star anise, turmeric, vanilla

Raw Dairy

Okay, dairy is not technically Paleo, since before agriculture began, no one would have consumed dairy after weaning. Some Paleo authors believe that dairy is not healthy. Some think it is inflammatory for only some of the population. Some avoid it because it happens to spike their insulin. And others consume it, especially raw, particularly high-fat types, since it is mostly fat. That's because all of the studies that show unhealthy effects were done on non-raw, commercial mainstream, hormone-added, low-fat dairy. It is entirely possible that raw, high-fat dairy is healthy for many. Only you know whether you can tolerate it well.

Cheese, cream cheese, heavy whipping cream, kefir, sour cream, whole milk, yogurt

Staples to Keep on Hand

Ground beef, steaks, roasts, chicken breasts, wild-caught fish and shrimp, eggs, tuna, uncured bacon or other sugar-free pork

Onions, avocados, mushrooms, red peppers, zucchini, lettuce, spinach, asparagus, tomatoes, cucumbers, bags of frozen veggies

Berries, lemons, limes, apples, bags of frozen fruits

Coconut flour, almond meal/flour

Almonds, almond butter, walnuts, pecans, pine nuts

Coconut oil, butter, ghee, EVOO, lard

Coconut milk, chicken broth, bone broth

Tomato paste, diced tomatoes, no-sugar salsas, red and green

Minced garlic, kalamata olives, sea salt, coarse black pepper, other spices like cilantro (great detox), basil, chili powder, rosemary, oregano, and cumin

Dairy items (preferably raw) if you eat it: heavy whipping cream, feta cheese, cream cheese, and cheddar cheese

Paleo on the Cheap Checklist

Be Smart about Paying for Organic

I know that many of you are concerned about toxins such as pesticides in our produce, but you might not be able to buy everything organic to protect yourself, due to financial constraints. If you can't buy organic, know that you are still eating healthier than 90% of Americans when you simply make Paleo food selections for yourself and your family, instead of the Standard American Diet (SAD).

However, if you can afford to buy some of your food organic, consider selecting organic for these foods that have been measured to be the most contaminated with pesticide residues:

- Apples
- Celery
- Cherries
- Grapes (Imported)
- Lettuce
- Nectarines
- Peaches
- Pears
- Spinach
- Strawberries
- Bell Peppers

If you buy anything organic at all, the top three that you should make an organic choice would be **apples, celery, and strawberries**, which pose the worst risks.

If you can't buy most of your foods organic, then here's a list of those that you could consider buying non-organic, knowing that they are the least contaminated:

- Asparagus
- Avocados
- Bananas
- Broccoli
- Cabbage
- Cantaloupe (Domestic)
- Eggplant
- Grapefruit
- Kiwi Fruit
- Mangoes
- Mushrooms
- Onions
- Papayas
- Pineapples
- Sweet Potatoes
- Watermelon

Onions, asparagus, avocados, eggplant, mangoes, and pineapples are the safest to buy non-organic.

You may want to consider donating to the Environmental Working Group, which performs the analysis of the research upon which these lists are based. www.ewg.com They also have downloadable apps for your smartphone with these lists, http://www.ewg.org/foodnews/guide/ although they do contain non-Paleo foods in the full lists.

Plan to Save

Construct Your Monthly Spending Plan

Clarity is what you are striving for here, so that you know exactly where the money is going to go. That clear understanding will make it much easier to know if extras are really warranted or even possible when you are tempted later.

Know What You Have before Shopping

Designate a day for weekly menu planning. Start your Meal Planning session with a Refrigerator Inventory and Clean-Out. It's a natural hand-in-hand activity to do with meal planning, since you can plan to use the last of whatever is still good, or freeze it if you can't use it right away, further cutting down on waste. If you make this a normal routine that you follow on one day of the week (say, Saturday morning), it will become second nature to do this.

If you have a can of coconut milk sitting in your pantry, include that food in your meal plan for that week, even if you have to research recipes because you haven't eaten it before; maybe it's a new Paleo food you've discovered that you wouldn't have eaten when you were eating like most folks still do. You'll save money that week and ensure that the food doesn't go to waste. Don't forget the food in the freezer, which doesn't have an unlimited shelf life and will eventually go bad, just like items in the pantry.

Plan Weekly Menus before Shopping

Think about meals at home, meals at work, plan for special occasions that involve eating out. Just taking a little time to plan can save more money than you may think by limiting waste. After you have a plan, create your grocery list based on it. It doesn't have to be set in stone, so if you see kale on sale, and you had Swiss chard on your list, you can make an on-the-spot substitution in the store.

Finally, construct your prep list of which items need to be pre-prepared by washing and chopping so that you save time when you are ready to cook. Cooking the night before or prepping the dish so that it's ready to pop in the oven the next morning can save you time, too; especially in the morning when you might not be awake enough to think of making breakfast.

You can even do batch cooking sessions once a month or once a week, so that your kitchen isn't heated up each day, which can increase utility costs. Cooking many dishes at once means that you are efficiently using your oven space, too, avoiding heating the oven for only one thing.

What you don't buy is important, too. Healthy food is found on the edges of the store, not usually in the middle of the store.

Don't go shopping when you are hungry. It will make it more difficult to stick to the list you made. Remember to use that membership card when going to the regular grocery store.

Use Chapter 4 to learn how to make your own convenience foods, thus cutting the grocery costs down even more.

If you plan simple meals, you just need a protein source, veggies, and a good fat for each one. Here's a weekly meal planning template with space for a grocery list for you to print out each week for your planning session:

http://tinyurl.com/wmptemp

Watch for Sales and Use Coupons

Use coupons or ask for a rain check and buy in large quantities when something Paleo goes on sale. For example, coconut oil is more expensive in local stores, but could be on sale online in larger quantities, for those things that don't spoil quickly. Or for those really-well-liked foods that you "consume in mass quantities" like the Coneheads from Saturday Night Live always did for their meals (I may be giving away my age here).

Store brands are often private-labeled from major suppliers, so give them a try to see if they provide the same quality at a lower price. You may be surprised.

Reduce Meat Costs the Smart Way

You don't have to pay top dollar for your protein to get top quality. Some simple ways to cut that expense down to size are:

Buy whole meat or poultry and cut it up yourself for $1 per pound savings over pre-cut.

Shop the section of meats that are reduced for quick sale due to expiration dates looming. Either cook it that day or freeze.

Eat Organic Organs and Offal

Buy and eat organic organs and offal, which are often healthier and always a cheaper cut of meat, because buyers are less familiar with them, or really do consider them "offal." Non-organic organ meat is more likely to contain toxins, antibiotics, or hormones, so this is one thing that you will want to buy organic if at all possible. Thrifty cuts like ox tail, tongue, beef liver, sweetbreads, chicken liver, kidneys, marrow, hocks, and hearts are delicious with the right recipes, and unbelievably cheap. Take my challenge to try a different organ or offal choice once a week with an excellent recipe to see if you become a fan of organ meats.

Roasts, shanks, shoulders, and stew meat also cost less than steaks and chops. Just cook these less expensive organs and thrift cuts in a liquid on low heat (a crockpot is a natural for this), and they will become much more tender. You can use the bones for broth or stock. If you can't normally buy grass-fed meats, organs are a great bargain that you CAN afford to buy grass-fed. For example, grass feed beef liver is $2-3 a pound and chicken livers are even cheaper than that, at $1-2 a pound. Pâté is worth the preparation time. As long as you are buying quality meat, organ meats are more nutritious than the more popular cuts, and eating "nose-to-tail" is even more Paleo!

27

Learn to Fish or Hunt

Take up a new hobby or form of relaxation and getting away from it all. This would have the added benefit of bringing you even closer to your food source, and you might be surprised at how much you enjoy it.

Befriend a Hunter or Fisher

If you would not enjoy the sport, you can always ask a buddy that does, if you could buy some of his or her hunting or fishing results.

Try Bulk Meat Buying

Cow pooling, in which you would contribute money in a common fund with others to buy meat in bulk, or just buying half a cow, bison, or lamb for your family can net you awesome savings on the healthiest meat. Yes, it is a lot of money to outlay all at once, but if you can swing it, this way of getting grass-fed beef is the least expensive in the long run. It will also give you a chance to try all the cuts of an animal, rather than eating only the cuts you are familiar with. New techniques and tastes are a definite advantage here.

If You Can't Buy Organic Meat…

You can protect yourself from antibiotics and hormones by avoiding fat from that source. If you will buy only leaner cuts, you can keep from getting the biggest dose of antibiotics, hormones, toxins, and Omega-6 pro-inflammatory fatty acids, which are stored in the fat. If you can't get lean cuts, then trim the fat before cooking. Same goes for the skin of mainstream chicken, for the same reasons. Beef, lamb, elk, bison (buffalo), goat, and venison are ruminants, which have access to a natural diet for at least some part of their lives, and therefore would have a more beneficial Omega-6 to Omega-3 balance than would chicken or pork.

Never Pay Retail For Organic Produce

Plant Your Own Garden

It's easier than you think, even on an apartment patio or balcony. Plant some berry bushes in the spring: strawberry, blueberry, blackberry, or cranberry. Being outside more tending to your garden will have the added benefit of ensuring that you get your daily dose of Vitamin D and connect with nature more.

Pick Your Own Produce

In season, you can go to a local orchard that allows you to pick-your-own fresh fruits. You can also be on the lookout for wild berries growing – a true gift from nature.

Join a Farm Share or CSA (Community-Supported Agriculture Program)

These are options that allow you to directly support your local farmers, without which you wouldn't have fresh quality produce. Use the links in the Appendix of this book to locate a local one.

Get to Know Your Local Farmers as Friends

Visit your local farmer's market in order to not only buy local, but also to make new friends. As a frequent customer, you will get to be known and recognized by them, which can have some side benefits. They might even give you some of the less popular items such as bones, organs, or fat for free as a gift for being such a loyal customer, if you let them know that you would welcome such.

Try the Farmer's Market at the End of the Day

Rather than take leftover produce home or have them go to waste, they may discount them for a quick sale if you are still hanging around then.

Render Your Own Fats

Buy fat from local farmers and render it yourself to make lard, suet, and tallow for pennies on the dollar. Pork, duck, beef, or lamb fat from your butcher or farmer's market will be very inexpensive because so few people ask for it or want it. You might need to ask the week before, but you can probably get these fats pretty easily and affordably. Supplementing your coconut oil, butter, and extra virgin olive oil with these animal fats is very Paleo and very cheap.

Consider a Few Equipment Purchases

Invest in equipment necessary to save you money in the long run, like a pressure cooker, crock pot, or dehydrator. These investments will also save you time, which usually ends up saving you money, too.

Using a pressure cooker saves both time and money because you don't heat up the house in the warm seasons when you are paying to keep the house cool. Items that would take hours in the oven or on the stove, take only minutes to cook in a pressure cooker, using the utilities for a shorter amount of time as well. This one is self-contained so that you don't even need a stove! Set it and forget it. http://tinyurl.com/digprescook

A crockpot can make cheaper cuts of meat tender, allowing you to save. You will probably want a programmable one that can travel easily in case you are going to a Paleo Potluck. http://tinyurl.com/crockpt1 http://tinyurl.com/crockpt2

Dehydrators are great for drying your own herbs, fruit, jerky, or making veggie chips for dipping. Kale chips are delicious! http://tinyurl.com/dehydrator1 http://tinyurl.com/dehydrator2

Use Your Freezer to Your Full Advantage

Buy a used freezer on Craig's List for under $100 to help you take advantage of bulk buys. If you are a member of a CSA or co-op and can't eat all the produce you receive, preserve it by canning, or freeze it after blanching, for those things that will freeze well.

If you are limited on freezer space and don't have room for a separate freezer, be friendly and split that cow or portion of a cow from a local farmer with a friend or another family.

Dehydrate, ferment, or freeze food that can't be used before it spoils. For example, turn cabbage into sauerkraut and fruit into dried fruit leather. Having frozen food available anytime you need it saves a trip to the store, saving gas. Frozen fruits and vegetables may not be optimal, but often can save money due to less waste. Buying fresh and blanching/freezing yourself is another option.

Vacuum Sealers Keep Food Fresh Longer

Vacuum-pack individual meat portions so that you can pull one out of the freezer when you need it. Cooked food takes up less space in the freezer than raw frozen foods, meaning that you make maximum use of your space. Zippered freezer bags will also work for shorter times. http://tinyurl.com/foodsaver1 http://tinyurl.com/foodsaver2

Buy Everything You Can In Bulk

Costco, Sam's, Trader Joe's, farmer's markets, co-ops, u-pick-it farms, wholesalers, or a grass-fed cow share will allow you to save on healthy food. Buy as close to the source as you can, to cut out the middle man and get the best deal possible. If you can find local farms, you get fresher, probably organic even if not certified organic, and you save the mark-up from transportation costs.

Even your neighborhood grocery store will have a natural foods or organic section. Spices that are not irradiated can be found in bulk (you can buy only as much as you want) at HEB in the natural foods section. And they are WAY cheaper than the pre-packaged spices in the regular spice isle. I got the same amount as in a small bottle of basil for a nickel.

Olive oil, for instance, is much less expensive when bought in gallon jugs than in the smaller glass bottles. Another good example would be ghee, which keeps a long time even at room temperature. This will also ensure that you shop less often to save gasoline, wear and tear on the vehicle, and your time.

Warehouse Stores and Online Bargains

Costco Paleo Items

A membership to Costco can more than pay for itself with regard to Paleo foods. Here's a list of what I found there:

- Organic Kirkland Beef, sourced from Verde Farms, which is also grass-fed. Depending upon your area, the source could be different. According to Costco Connection magazine, beef is sourced from the US, Canada, or Australia. Australian cattle sources are 100 percent organic grass-fed. About half of the US and Canadian animals are 100% grass-fed, but the other half is organic grain-finished. 4 lbs. for $17.99

- American Organic Grass-Fed Tenderloin Steaks $13.89 per lb.

- Australian/NZ Free-Range and Grass-fed Lamb Leg: $4.99 per lb. Rack: $11.99 per lb. Loin Chop: $7.99 per lb.

- Kirkland Low-Sodium Sliced Bacon 4 lb. $10.99

- Jones All Natural Uncured Canadian Bacon 24 oz. $10.99

- Coleman Natural Uncured Beef Hot Dogs 3 lb. $10.99

- High Plains 100% Bison Hot Dogs Uncured (No Hormones or Antibiotics) $15.99 for 1.73 lb.

- Eggs 15 Dozen $15.69

- Organic Kirkland Pastured Cage-Free Brown Eggs 2 Dozen $6.39

- 24-Pack of Almark Hard Boiled Eggs $4.35

- Organic Ground Turkey $4.99 per lb.

- Coleman Organic Whole Chicken $2.29 per lb.

- Coleman Organic Chicken Breast $5.99 per lb.

- Coleman Organic Chicken Thighs $3.99 per lb.

- Pacific Organic Chicken Broth 6 x 32 oz. $10.99

- Kirkland Chicken Stock 6 x 32 oz. $8.95

- Kirkland Wild-Caught Smoked Salmon 2 x 8 oz. $15.59

- Frozen Wild-Caught Cooked and Peeled Langostino Lobster Tails 2 lb. for $22.99

  Frozen Wild-Caught Lobster Tails $17.25 per lb.

- Frozen Wild-Caught Mahi Mahi 3 lb. $19.39

- Frozen Wild-Caught Mahi Mahi Burgers 3 lb. $15.99

- Frozen Wild-Caught Ahi Tuna Steak 3 lb. $29.99

- Frozen Kirkland Wild-Caught Alaskan Pacific Cod Filets 2 lb. $15.99

- Frozen Kirkland Wild-Caught Hake Loins 2.5 lb. $13.99

- Frozen Kirkland Wild-Caught Alaskan Sockeye Salmon 2.5 lb $18.49

- Fresh Wild-Caught Sockeye Salmon $8.99 per lb.

- Bear and Wolf Wild-Caught Canned Salmon 6 – 6 oz. $10.99

- Frozen Kirkland Wild-Caught Scallops 2 lb. $26.99

- Season Tinned Sardines In Olive Oil 5 – 3.75 oz. $7.99

- Kirkland Organic Butter 2 lb. $7.99

- Kerrygold Pastured Butter

- Kerrygold Pastured Cheese (Reserve Cheddar and Dubliner)

- President Feta Cheese (both crumbled and block)

- Kirkland Shredded Mexican Blend Cheese 2.5 lb. $5.99

- Raskas Cream Cheese 3 lb. $5.59

- Promised Land Heavy Cream 32 oz. $3.29

- Kirkland Organic Low-fat Milk 3 x 64 oz $9.99

- Kirkland Organic Whole Milk 3 x 64 oz $10.99

- Flax Milk 6 – 32 oz. $11.49

- Unsweetened Almond Milk 6 – 32 oz. $9.99

- Zico Coconut Water 24 x 14 oz. $17.99

- Rita Coco Coconut Water 6 x 1 Liter $14.99

- Large Wholly Guacamole $9.49

- Rojo's Fresh Pico de Gallo 48 oz. $5.49

- Fresh Gourmet Jack's Special Salsa 48 oz. Jar $5.45

- Alexia Frozen Sweet Potato Fries 4 lb. $6.59

- Frozen Organic Broccoli 4 lb. $5.89

- Bella Sun Luci Sun-Dried Tomatoes Jar 32 oz. $7.99

- Organic Baby Spinach and Organic Spring Mix

- Organic Canned Tomato Sauce 12 – 15 oz. $7.69

- Organic Canned Tomato Paste 12 – 6 oz. $6.39

- Organic Canned Diced Tomatoes 8 – 14 oz. $7.69

- Organic Canned Stewed Tomatoes 8 – 14 oz. $7.69

- Organic Mashups Squeezable Fruit 12 Pouches $9.99

- Ro-Tel Diced Tomatoes and Green Chiles 8 x 10 oz. $6.49

- Kirkland Dried Cherries 20 oz. $6.99

- Kirkland Dried Blueberries 20 oz. $9.89

- Frozen Organic Wild Blueberries 4 lb. $14.79

- Pre-Cut Organic Apples 8 x 6 oz. Bags $7.99

- Azuma Calamari Salad 24 oz. $11.79

- Nikko Sesame Seaweed Salad 16 oz. $6.69

- Krinos Kalamata Olives 32 oz. $6.59

- Carbonell Queen Green Olives 2 – 21 oz. $6.95

- Lindsay Ripe Olives 33 oz. Foil Pack $3.49

- Larabars Variety Pack 18 ct. $15.85

- Kirkland Marinara Sauce Jar (No Additives or Sugar) 3 x 32 oz. $5.99

- Classico Tomato & Basil Spaghetti Sauce Jar (No Additives or Sugar) 3 x 32 oz. $7.49

- Kirkland Organic Extra Virgin Olive Oil 1.5 Liter $8.99

- Belolio Grapeseed Oil 2 liter $8.69

- UTZ Pork Rinds Barrel 18 oz. $5.99

- Kirkland Walnuts 48 oz. $17.99

- Kirkland Pistachios 48 oz. $15.69

- Kirkland Pine Nuts 24 oz. $17.59

- Kirkland Pecan Halves 32 oz. $15.99

- Kirkland Almonds (soak/dehydrate, make almond meal or flour) 48 oz. $10.89

- Mariani Sliced Premium Almonds 32 oz. $7.99

- MaraNatha All Natural Creamy Almond Butter 26. Oz. $5.99

- Kirkland Brands Green Tea Matcha Blend 100 ct. $14.99

- Ruta Maya 100% Organic Coffee 2.2 lb. $14.99

- Kirkland Brand Real 100% Maple Syrup 32 oz. $12.99

- Nature Nate's Raw Unfiltered Honey 40 oz. $13.95

- Purevia Stevia Natural Sweetener 800 ct. $15.99

- Kirkland Minced Fresh Garlic 48 oz. $3.99

- Chef Cuisine Peeled Garlic 3 lb. $4.99

- Terra Sweet Potato Chips 16.5 oz. $5.89

- Seasoned Roasted Seaweed 10 Bags $8.99

- Frankly Fresh Rice/Tomato Grape Leaves Wraps 32 oz. $10.59

- Sukhi's Chicken Tikka Masala 32 oz. $10.99

- Ready-Made Chicken Korma, (Caramel Color, Though)

- Alaskan Wild Salmon Oil 150 ct. 1000 mg. $16.89

- Kirkland Fish Oil 400 ct. 1000 mg. $7.99

- Nature's Bounty Fish Oil 130 ct. 1400 mg. $19.89

- Schiff Mega Red Krill Oil 300 mg. 90 ct. $18.49

- Schiff Mega Red Krill Oil Extra Strength $18.49

- Ubiquinol Co-Q-10 100 mg. ct. $34.99

- Vitamin D (2000 IU $10.89 and 5000 IU $16.99)

- Kirkland Freeze-Dried Fruit No Sugar Added 20 x 10-12 gram pouches $13.69

- Fruit Leather Strips No Sugar Added 48 x .5 oz. $10.59

- Paleo Comfort Foods Cookbook $18.99

- Everyday Paleo Cookbook $18.99

Sam's Club Paleo Items

A Sam's Club membership might not be quite as valuable with regard to Paleo foods, but here is a list of what I found there:

- Zia Fresh Bratwurst 5 lb. $13.48

- 80/20 Ground Chuck $2.98 Per Pound

- Wild-Caught Scallops 2 lb. $25.98

- Wild-Caught Cod Loins 2.5 lb. $13.88

- Wild-Caught Sockeye Salmon 2.5 lb. $24.98

- Wild-Caught Alaskan Flounder Fillets 3 lb. $11.98

- Wild-Caught Salmon 1.875 $15.98

- SeaPak Salmon Burgers 2.5 lb. $14.98

- Honey Boy Wild-Caught Canned Salmon 4 x 14.75 oz. $9.88

- Eggs 15 Dozen $15.69

- Brown Cage-Free Eggs 1.5 Dozen $3.23

- Eggland's Best Eggs 1.5 Dozen $3.38

- Kerrygold Butter $7.50 2 lb.

- Kerrygold Cheeses (Ballyshannon and Dubliner) $5.50 Per Pound

- Kerrygold Dubliner Cheese Snacks 30 count .6 oz. Bars $9.99

- Biazzo Whole Milk Ricotta Cheese $5.73

- Greek Isle Crumbled Feta $7.48

- Greek Isle Flavored Crumbled Feta $8.66

- Salemville Amish Blue Cheese Crumbles $9.47

- Horizon Organic 2% Milk 3 – Half Gallons $10.98

- Daisy Sour Cream 3 lb. $3.99

- Land O' Lakes Whipping Cream 32 oz. $3.35

- Silk Almond Milk 3 x Half Gallons $7.98

- Organic Spring Mix 1 lb. $3.90

- Organic Spinach 1 lb. $4.48

- Wholly Guacamole 36 oz. $8.98

- Member's Mark Extra Virgin Olive Oil 3 liter $14.58

- Italian Rose Fresh Salsa 48 oz. $6.98

- Artisan Fresh Bruschetta $7.48

- 60% Cacao 3 lb. Ghirardelli Bittersweet Chocolate Chips $9.48

- Larabars Variety Pack 18 ct. $13.01

- Classico Tomato & Basil Spaghetti Sauce Jar (No Additives or Sugar) 3 x 32 oz. $7.48

- Spice World Fresh Minced Garlic 48 oz. $3.90

- MaraNatha All Natural Creamy Almond Butter 26 oz. $6.28

- Daily Chef Raw Whole Almonds 48 ox. $10.98

- Diamond Sliced Almonds 32 oz. $7.98

- Diamond Walnuts 32 oz. $11.74

- Young's Raw Pecan Halves 32 oz. $15.87

- Salt and Pepper Pistachios 24 oz. $8.98

- Uncle Luke's 100% Maple Syrup 32 oz. $13.28

- Mario Green Olives 2 x 21 oz. $5.98

- Mario Queen Green Olives 2 x 21 oz. $6.98

- Early California Ripe Pitted Olives 6 x 6 oz. $6.78

- Lipton Cold Brew Family Size Tea Bags 66 ct. $6.88

- Simply Right Stevia 200 ct. $9.98

- Simply Right Vitamin D 2000 IU 400 ct. $8.48

- Simply Right Vitamin D 5000 IU 400 ct. $9.98

- Simply Right Vitamin D 10000 IU 400 ct. $8.81

- Mega Red Krill Oil 300 mg. 90 ct. $18.56

- Simply Right Co-Q-10 100 mg. 180 ct. $15.98

- Simply Right Co-Q-10 200 mg. 120 ct. $23.98

- Simply Right Co-Q-10 400 mg. 60 ct. $29.98

Amazon Paleo Items

I don't know how I lived without Amazon Prime for so long. It gives you free two-day shipping on many (but not all) Amazon items, with no minimum order. After the initial free trial, Amazon Prime is $79 annually. http://tinyurl.com/AmPrime

If you have a college email address, you can get Amazon Prime for free for six months through Amazon Student: http://tinyurl.com/AmStudent. If you are a member of the Amazon Mom program, you can also get it for free at first: http://tinyurl.com/AmaMom.

If you have the paid version, you also get unlimited instant streaming of thousands of movies and TV shows, as well as the ability to borrow a Kindle book for free each month from the Kindle Owners' Lending Library.

Another Amazon program that I love for repeat periodic purchases is Subscribe and Save, which gives you an extra 5-15% off and Free Shipping if you don't have Amazon Prime already. You can set the frequency to as long as 6 months and can delay any shipment when they notify you by email that the next shipment is going to be sent, if you don't need more then. Here's a list of items that are eligible for Subscribe and Save:

Amazon offers the Wild Planet line of seafood products, which are some of the best canned seafood available, with no BPA, Wild/ Sustainable, and no MSG.

Wild Planet Wild Sardines in Extra Virgin Olive Oil, 4.375-Ounce (Pack of 6) $13.52 http://tinyurl.com/WPSardines

Wild Planet Sustainably Caught Wild Albacore Tuna, 5 Ounce Cans (Pack of 6) $12.70 http://tinyurl.com/WPTuna

Wild Planet Sustainably Caught Wild Skipjack Light Tuna, 5 Ounce Cans (Pack of 12) $21.13 http://tinyurl.com/WPTuna2

Wild Planet Wild Alaskan Sockeye Salmon, Skinless & Boneless, 6 Ounce Can (Pack of 4) $15.59 http://tinyurl.com/WPSalmon

Nanak Pure Desi Ghee, Clarified Butter, 28-Ounce Jar $13.07 http://tinyurl.com/NanakGhee

Emerald Cove Instant Pacific Sea Salad (Six Varieties of Sea Vegetables), 0.75-Ounce Bags (Pack of 6) $28.70 http://tinyurl.com/SeaVegs

Nutiva Organic Extra Virgin Coconut Oil, 15-Ounce Tubs (Pack of 2) $14.81 http://tinyurl.com/OEVCO1

Zoe Organic Extra Virgin Olive Oil, 25.5-Ounce Tins (Pack of 2) $21.48 http://tinyurl.com/OEVOO1

Caribbean Joy Coconut Milk, 13.5-Ounce (Pack of 24) $30.05 http://tinyurl.com/CocoMilk1

Let's Do Organic Creamed Coconut, 7-Ounce Boxes (Pack of 6) $11.63 http://tinyurl.com/CreamCoco

Let's Do Organic Shredded, Unsweetened Coconut, 8-Ounce Packages (Pack of 12) $20.15 Use this for crusting chicken, beef, or shrimp, when you're feeling desperate for some "breaded" fried comfort food http://tinyurl.com/ShredCoco

Bob's Red Mill Organic Coconut Flour, 16-Ounce Units (Pack of 4) $22.51 http://tinyurl.com/CocoFlour1

Bob's Red Mill Almond Meal/Flour, 16-Ounce Packages (Pack of 4) $30.50 http://tinyurl.com/AlmondFlour1

Justin's Nut Butter Natural Maple Almond Butter, 16-Ounce Plastic Jar (Pack of 3) $22.16 http://tinyurl.com/AlmondButter

Justin's Nut Butter Natural Classic Almond Butter 10 Count Squeeze Packs, 11.5-Ounce Boxes (Pack of 3) $21.42 These are good for easy portion control since a packet is about 200 calories.http://tinyurl.com/AlmondButter2

Mauna Loa Macadamias, Dry Roasted with Sea Salt, 4.5-Ounce Containers (Pack of 4) $21.37 http://tinyurl.com/MacaNuts

Homemade Dressing Mix Variety Pack (French Garden, Napa Garden & Italian Garden), 3.3 to 4-Ounce Containers I love these mixes for quick spices to use in salad dressings. http://tinyurl.com/HomemadeDressingMix

Farmer's Market Foods Organic Butternut Squash, 15-Ounce Cans (Pack of 12) $24.07 http://tinyurl.com/ButternutSquash1

Madhava Honey Stix, Pure Natural Clover Honey, 100-Count Jars (Pack of 2) $29.19 Honey Straws 4.3 g Carbs
http://tinyurl.com/HoneyStix

Great Lakes Select Honey, Clover, 32-Ounce Bottles (Pack of 3) $14.76 This one is not from any countries that sell or import the fake corn syrup "honey" from China.
http://tinyurl.com/SelectHoney

Coombs Family Farms 100% Pure Maple Syrup Premium Grade B, 32-Ounce Bear Jug $17.31
http://tinyurl.com/MapleSyrup1

Good Sense Omega Munchies, Caramelized Flaxseed Walnuts, Maple, 5-Ounce Bags (Pack of 6) $16.42
http://tinyurl.com/OmegaMunch

Bare Fruit 100% Organic Bake-Dried Apples, Fuji, 1 Pound Bags (Pack of 2) $15.63 http://tinyurl.com/BDApples

Funky Monkey Snacks Bananamon, 0.42-Ounce Bags (Pack of 12) $8.87 Crunchy dried fruit
http://tinyurl.com/Bananamon

Navitas Naturals Cacao Powder, 16-Ounce Pouches (Pack of 2) $23.34 http://tinyurl.com/CacaoPowder1

Navitas Naturals Cacao Nibs, 16-Ounce Pouches (Pack of 2) $23.85 http://tinyurl.com/CacaoNibs1

Go Raw Freeland Flax Snax, Pizza Flax Snax, 3.0-Ounce Bags (Pack of 6) $19.53 http://tinyurl.com/FlaxSnax

Lowrey's Bacon Curls, Microwave Pork Rinds (Chicharrones) $16.14 http://tinyurl.com/MWBRinds

Zevia All Natural Soda, Ginger Ale, 12-Ounce Cans (Pack of 24) sweetened with erythritol/stevia $16.63
http://tinyurl.com/ZeviaSoda

Lipton Iced Tea, 48-Count Gallon SizeTea Bags $14.26
http://tinyurl.com/LiptonGallonBags

These next two would be for an occasional indulgence under the 80/20 rule (hey, at least there's no wheat belly wheat):

Chebe Bread Pizza Crust Mix, Gluten Free, 7.5-Ounce Box (Pack of 8) $18.16 http://tinyurl.com/GFPizzaCrust

Pamela's Ultimate Gluten-Free Baking and Pancake Mix, 4-Pound Bags (Pack of 3) $37.92
http://tinyurl.com/GFBakingMix

The next few items are not Subscribe and Save, but you may be interested anyway, since they are hard-to-find items.

Foods Alive Golden Flax Crackers, Regular, 4-Ounce Pouches (Pack of 6) $26.95 http://tinyurl.com/FlaxCrax

Foods Alive Golden Flax Crackers, Onion Garlic, 4-Ounce Pouches (Pack of 6) $26.95 http://tinyurl.com/OGFlax

Mae Ploy Thai Red Curry Paste - 14 ounce per jar $5.97
http://tinyurl.com/ThaiRCurry

San J Organic Wheat Free Tamari Soy Sauce Gold Label Travel Packs, 200-Count Packages $23.08
http://tinyurl.com/GFTamari

Avoid Spoiled Produce and Other Waste

A 2010 report from the U.S. Bureau of Applied Research in Anthropology revealed that an average of $590 is wasted by a family of four every year on food they throw out. Total, approximately $43 billion annually in the U.S. goes in the trash. Yet another 2010 University of Arizona study showed that each year, an average American household discards fourteen percent of the food purchased, 15% of which is unexpired and unopened.

Fifty to a hundred years ago, just about everybody knew how to "waste not, want not." Efficiency with any resource was built into most tasks, including the knowledge of how to make everything last and serve its purpose, most especially food. Let's bring back that wisdom today.

Don't throw away bones, pan drippings, or other leftovers. Save the bones to make bone broth or stock (See Chapter 4). Pan drippings can be used for flavoring veggies and adding that essential Paleo fat serving to them.

Use the green bags made with zeolite that absorb ethylene to cut down on produce spoilage. Each bag can be reused at least ten times. Never refrigerate wet produce. Let dry first. http://tinyurl.com/greenbagset

To keep potatoes longer, take them out of the bag. Throw away any that already have spots. Wash and dry the rest to remove any mold or fungi. This can increase the time they last from days to months.

Alternatively, you can store potatoes, turnips, parsnips, rutabagas, and other root vegetables in sand in large containers under burlap sacks in your cellar, after first sorting, washing, and drying as described previously.

Get a Baggy Rack that props up the zippered plastic bags so that you can fill them easily yourself. You can get 4 of them (enough to gift one or two to someone you love) for $16.19: http://tinyurl.com/baggyracks

Another convenience tool for Paleo folks, who deal with lots of produce, is the Scrap Trap, for quickly sliding scraps into a container that attaches to your drawer or cabinet door, with the scraping tool included that handily fits right in it. $7.78 http://tinyurl.com/scraptraps

Which Produce Needs to Be Eaten First?

If you consult these charts before deciding what to cook and serve, it can substantially reduce the amount of money wasted on spoiled produce. Average times that produce can be safely stored in both refrigerator and freezer are given, allowing you to make smart choices in meal planning. Foods are listed in order of most perishable foods, so that you can use them first.

Fruits and Vegetables by Spoils First

Fruit/Vegetable	Refrigerator	Freezer
Yucca (Cassava)	1-2 days	8-12 months
Currants	1-2 days	8-12 months
Figs	2-3 days	8-12 months
Persimmons	2-3 days	8-12 months
Berries	2-3 days	8-12 months
Cherries	2-3 days	8-12 months
Pineapples	2-3 days	4-6 months
Asparagus	2-3 days	8-12 months
Bok Choy	2-3 days	8-12 months
Cilantro	2-3 days	8-12 months
Kohlrabi (leaves)	2-3 days	8-12 months
Cherimoyas	2-5 days RT	8-12 months
Guavas	2-5 days RT	8-12 months
Papayas	2-5 days RT	8-12 months
Bananas	2-5 days RT	8-12 months
Mangoes	2-5 days RT	8-12 months
Plantains	3-5 days RT	8-12 months
Purslane	3-5 days	4-6 months
Apricots	3-5 days	8-12 months
Avocados	3-5 days	8-12 months
Grapes	3-5 days	8-12 months
Kiwis (Chinese Gooseberry)	3-5 days	4-6 months
Nectarines	3-5 days	8-12 months
Peaches	3-5 days	8-12 months
Pears	3-5 days	8-12 months

Fruit/Vegetable	Refrigerator	Freezer
Plums	3-5 days	8-12 months
Okra	3-5 days	NR
Rhubarb	3-5 days	NR
Broccoli	3-5 days	8-12 months
Brussels Sprouts	3-5 days	8-12 months
Greens (Collards, Swiss Chard, Kale, Mustard, Turnip, etc.)	3-5 days	8-12 months
Squash, summer	3-5 days	8-12 months
Zucchini	3-5 days	8-12 months
Cucumber	4-5 days	NR
Yam	1 week RT	8-12 months
Lychees	1 week	8-12 months
Passion Fruit	1 week	8-12 months
Star Fruit (Carambola)	1 week	8-12 months
Melons	1 week	8-12 months
Mushrooms	1 week	8-12 months
Chilies	1 week	NR
Lettuce	1 week	NR
Spinach	1 week	NR
Artichokes	1 week	8-12 months
Cauliflower	1 week	8-12 months
Eggplant	1 week	8-12 months
Kohlrabi (stems)	1 week	8-12 months
Leek	1 week	8-12 months
Peppers	1 week	8-12 months
Tomatillos	1 week	8-12 months
Tomatoes	1 week	8-12 months
Onions, green	1-2 weeks	NR
Cabbage	1-2 weeks	NR
Celery	2 weeks	8-12 months
Pomegranates	2 weeks	8-12 months
Citrus Fruits	2 weeks	4-6 months
Cantaloupe	2 weeks	8-12 months
Turnips	2 weeks	8-12 months

Fruit/Vegetable	Refrigerator	Freezer
Green Beans	2 weeks	NR
Parsley	2 weeks	NR
Radishes	2 weeks	NR
Beets	2 weeks	8-12 months
Carrots	2 weeks	8-12 months
Parsnips	2 weeks	8-12 months
Squash, winter	2 weeks	8-12 months
Jicama	2-3 weeks	8-12 months
Nopales	3 weeks	NR
Sweet Potatoes	3 weeks RT	8-12 months
Apples	1 month	8-12 months
Onions, yellow, white, red	1-2 months RT	8-12 months
Rutabagas	2 months	8-12 months

RT= Room Temperature

NR = Not Recommended

Fruits and Vegetables in Alpha Order

Fruit/Vegetable	Refrigerator	Freezer
Apples	1 month	8-12 months
Apricots	3-5 days	8-12 months
Artichokes	1 week	8-12 months
Asparagus	2-3 days	8-12 months
Avocados	3-5 days	8-12 months
Bananas	2-5 days RT	8-12 months
Beets	2 weeks	8-12 months
Berries	2-3 days	8-12 months
Bok Choy	2-3 days	8-12 months
Broccoli	3-5 days	8-12 months
Brussels Sprouts	3-5 days	8-12 months
Cabbage	1-2 weeks	NR
Cantaloupe	2 weeks	8-12 months
Carrots	2 weeks	8-12 months
Cauliflower	1 week	8-12 months

Fruit/Vegetable	Refrigerator	Freezer
Celery	2 weeks	8-12 months
Cherimoyas	2-5 days RT	8-12 months
Cherries	2-3 days	8-12 months
Chilies	1 week	NR
Cilantro	2-3 days	8-12 months
Citrus Fruits	2 weeks	4-6 months
Cucumber	4-5 days	NR
Currants	1-2 days	8-12 months
Eggplant	1 week	8-12 months
Figs	2-3 days	8-12 months
Grapes	3-5 days	8-12 months
Green Beans	2 weeks	NR
Greens (Collards, Swiss Chard, Kale, Mustard, Turnip, etc.)	3-5 days	8-12 months
Guavas	2-5 days RT	8-12 months
Jicama	2-3 weeks	8-12 months
Kiwis (Chinese Gooseberry)	3-5 days	4-6 months
Kohlrabi (leaves)	2-3 days	8-12 months
Kohlrabi (stems)	1 week	8-12 months
Leek	1 week	8-12 months
Lettuce	1 week	NR
Lychees	1 week	8-12 months
Mangoes	2-5 days RT	8-12 months
Melons	1 week	8-12 months
Mushrooms	1 week	8-12 months
Nectarines	3-5 days	8-12 months
Nopales	3 weeks	NR
Okra	3-5 days	NR
Onions, green	1-2 weeks	NR
Onions, yellow, white, red	1-2 months RT	8-12 months
Papayas	2-5 days RT	8-12 months
Parsley	2 weeks	NR
Parsnips	2 weeks	8-12 months

Fruit/Vegetable	Refrigerator	Freezer
Passion Fruit	1 week	8-12 months
Peaches	3-5 days	8-12 months
Pears	3-5 days	8-12 months
Peppers	1 week	8-12 months
Persimmons	2-3 days	8-12 months
Pineapples	2-3 days	4-6 months
Plantains	3-5 days RT	8-12 months
Plums	3-5 days	8-12 months
Pomegranates	2 weeks	8-12 months
Purslane	3-5 days	4-6 months
Radishes	2 weeks	NR
Rhubarb	3-5 days	NR
Rutabagas	2 months	8-12 months
Spinach	1 week	NR
Squash, summer	3-5 days	8-12 months
Squash, winter	2 weeks	8-12 months
Star Fruit (Carambola)	1 week	8-12 months
Sweet Potatoes	3 weeks RT	8-12 months
Tomatillos	1 week	8-12 months
Tomatoes	1 week	8-12 months
Turnips	2 weeks	8-12 months
Yam	1 week RT	8-12 months
Yucca (Cassava)	1-2 days	8-12 months
Zucchini	3-5 days	8-12 months

RT= Room Temperature

NR = Not Recommended

When to Eat What

You need to know which produce will spoil first, so that nothing goes to waste. Let's say that you go shopping on Saturday each week. In that case, these items need to be eaten Sunday to Monday because they only last 1-2 days:

- Yucca (Cassava)

- Currants

This list should be eaten next, up until Tuesday:

- Asparagus
- Berries
- Bok Choy
- Cherries
- Cilantro
- Figs
- Kohlrabi (leaves)
- Persimmons
- Pineapples

Next, eat these items that stay fresh up to 5 days, by Thursday:

- Cherimoyas
- Guava
- Papaya
- Bananas
- Mangoes
- Plantains
- Purslane
- Apricots
- Avocados
- Grapes
- Kiwis (Chinese Gooseberry)
- Nectarines
- Peaches
- Pears
- Plums
- Rhubarb
- Okra
- Rhubarb
- Broccoli
- Brussels Sprouts

- Greens (Spinach, Collards, Swiss Chard, Kale, Mustard, Turnip, etc.)
- Squash, summer
- Zucchini
- Cucumber

Finally, eat these foods by Saturday:

- Mushrooms
- Yam
- Lychees
- Passion Fruit
- Star Fruit (Carambola)
- Melons
- Chilies
- Lettuce
- Spinach
- Artichokes
- Cauliflower
- Eggplant
- Kohlrabi (stems)
- Leek
- Peppers
- Tomatillos
- Tomatoes
- Onions, green
- Cabbage

This list can carry over to next week or next month if necessary:

- Celery
- Pomegranates
- Citrus Fruits (Lemons/Limes/Oranges/ Grapefruits)
- Cantaloupe
- Turnips
- Green Beans
- Parsley

- Radishes
- Beets
- Carrots
- Parsnips
- Squash, winter
- Jicama

This list can carry over to next week or next month if necessary:

- Nopales
- Sweet Potatoes
- Apples
- Onions, yellow, white, red
- Rutabagas

If you have reached the day when something should be eaten, but can't eat it right then, just freeze it in zippered or vacuum bags to avoid waste.

Which Foods Need to be Stored Away from Others

Foods that emit lots of ethylene (the colorless, odorless gaseous hormone that all fruits and veggies give of) include apples, apricots, avocados, unripe bananas, cantaloupe, cherimoya, figs, honeydews, nectarines, papaya, peaches, pears, plums, and tomatoes. Ethylene causes ripening.

Separate the list above from the next list, which are foods that are extra sensitive to the effects of ethylene. These include ripe bananas, broccoli, Brussels sprouts, cabbage, carrots, cauliflower, cucumbers, eggplant, kiwi, lettuce (and other leafy greens), parsley, peas, peppers, summer squash, sweet potatoes, and watermelon. You don't want these to spoil faster.

That's exactly why you've got two crisper drawers at a minimum in your refrigerator!

What to Store Where: A Handy Chart

^ **Ethylene producers (keep away from other fruits and vegetables)**

Ethylene sensitive (keep away from producers above)

* **Cold sensitive**

Store in Refrigerator	^ Apples (storage >7 days)
	^ Apricots
	^ Cantaloupe
	^ Figs
	^ Honeydew
	Artichokes
	Asparagus
	Beets
	Blackberries
	Blueberries
	Broccoli
	Brussels sprouts
	Cabbage
	Carrots
	Cauliflower
	Celery
	Cherries
	Corn
	Grapes
	Green beans
	Green onions
	Herbs (except basil)
	Lima beans
	Leafy vegetables
	Leeks
	Lettuce
	Mushrooms
	Okra
	Peas

	Plums Radishes Raspberries Spinach Sprouts Strawberries Summer squash Yellow squash Zucchini
Cold Sensitive (spoils faster in cold) **Store on Counter**	^ Apples (storage < 7 days) ^ *Bananas ^ *Tomatoes Basil Cucumbers Eggplant Garlic Ginger Grapefruit Jicama Lemons Limes Mangoes Melons Oranges Papayas Peppers Persimmons Pineapples Plantains Pomegranates Watermelon

Ripen on Counter at Room Temperature, Then Refrigerate When Ripe	# Kiwi * ^ Avocados * ^ Nectarines * ^ Peaches * ^ Pears * ^ Plums
Store in a Cool Dry Place – Only Refrigerate after Cutting Open	Garlic Onions (not near potatoes) Potatoes (not near onions) Sweet potatoes Winter Squash (acorn, butternut, spaghetti, pumpkin)

Refrigerate these ^ gas releasers:

^ Apples (after 7 days)
^ Apricots
^ Cantaloupe
^ Figs
^ Honeydew

Don't refrigerate these * cold sensitive ^ gas releasers until they are ripe, and then not for long, because for them cold accelerates spoilage:

* Avocados
* Bananas, unripe
* Nectarines
* Peaches
* Pears
* Plums
* Tomatoes

Keep these # Ethylene sensitive foods away from all gas releasers:

Asparagus
Bananas, ripe
Bok Choy
Broccoli
Brussels sprouts
Cabbage
Carrots
Cauliflower
Celery
Chard
Cucumbers
Eggplant
Green Beans
Guavas
Herbs
Kiwi
Leeks
Lettuce and other leafy greens
Mangoes
Mushrooms
Okra
Parsley
Parsnips
Peaches
Pears
Peas
Peppers
Persimmons
Plums
Squash
Sweet potatoes
Watermelon

Some vegetables need cool, dark, and dry. Never refrigerate these fresh produce items until they have been cut open:

Garlic
Onions (not near potatoes)
Potatoes (not near onions)
Sweet potatoes
Winter Squash (acorn, butternut, spaghetti, pumpkin, etc)

Some fruits and vegetables will last better at room temperature for the first 4 or 5 days while whole:

Melons
Pineapples
Peppers
Eggplant
Tomatoes
Cucumbers

Tips and Tricks for Keeping Food Fresh Longer

Any fruit or vegetable, especially berries, will last much longer if you use a vinegar rinse before you store them. Mix one part vinegar (white or apple cider) and ten parts water and swirl the produce in this liquid. Let the food air-dry for 10 minutes before storing in the fridge. The rinse works by killing mold and bacteria that might be on the fruits and vegetables, allowing them to last from one to two weeks instead of days, in the case of strawberries, for instance.

Use Vitamin C (ascorbic acid) powder for preserving apples, bananas, avocados, eggplant, and any other produce that browns after you cut it open. Sprinkle it on your fruits or guacamole and cover them tightly with plastic wrap. http://tinyurl.com/VCPowder Both will last days in the fridge when treated this way. Be aware that the powder does have a tangy, lemony taste. In some cases, you might want to dilute the ascorbic acid, such as storing apples in a mix of 1/2 teaspoon in 1 cup of water.

Another tip is to make sure your refrigerator's temperature is set between 34 and 39 degrees to preserve foods the longest.

Just separating the ethylene-producers from the ethylene sensitive produce as outlined in the previous sections will work wonders for reducing your produce waste.

Remove any leafy tops on produce before storing. They continue to draw in oxygen, encouraging faster oxidation and decay. For example, strawberries with the tops left on them will take on more oxygen through the green leaves than those with the tops removed, thus ripening and spoiling more quickly.

Do not wash before storing—moisture encourages spoilage.

Store in crisper or moisture-resistant bag or wrap. Consider using the green bags that retard spoilage further.

Wrap uncut cantaloupe and honeydew to prevent odor spreading to other foods.

Discard bruised or decayed fruit quickly.

Wrap cut surfaces of melon and citrus fruit to prevent Vitamin C loss.

Before serving leftovers, slice off 1/4 inch of the surface and discard. Bacteria accumulate in the cut surface.

By storing leftover foods in a container that fits exactly, you decrease the chances for spoilage because of less air being trapped in the container.

Ripen tomatoes at room temperature away from direct sunlight; then refrigerate. Eat as soon as possible, preferably before it even goes in the refrigerator, since cold will retard the enzymes that make the tomato taste best. Refrigerate all cut tomatoes after wrapping the cut edge, and use promptly.

Eating Paleo Saves on Other Expenses

These include the junk, processed foods, and snacks you used to eat, not to mention drugs and medical bills you won't have in the long run, which is a priceless savings in terms of your quality of life, especially as you get older. When you take that into consideration, you can see that you might not be spending that much more than before you went Paleo.

Paleo Frugal Food Friends (FFF)

Eggs are one of your FFFs that you need to get to know better. Using eggs to their full advantage will give you lots of savings over traditional meat, fish, or poultry protein selections. You can get even the best kinds of cage-free pastured organic eggs for less than most other protein sources.

Think of eggs the same way that Bubba thought about shrimp in the Forrest Gump movie: Hard-boiled, deviled, scrambled, soft-boiled, fried, huevos rancheros, omelets, scotch eggs, baked, soufflés, over easy, frittatas, heuvos con chorizo, steamed, egg foo young, poached, pocket eggs, pickled, egg salad, migas, crepes, sunny-side-up, shakshouka, quiche, ... the list goes on and on. When I did some research on this, I found that according to chef lore, the number of pleats or folds in a chef's hat used to represent the number of ways that the chef knew how to prepare eggs. And apparently, there are well over 100 ways to fix eggs, making them the Queen of Versatility.

Paleo Carbs can cut that food bill if you are at your ideal weight. If you eat more carbohydrates such as sweet potatoes, carrots, beets, yams, or even regular potatoes, you can save. Remember that seasonal produce is better for you, and always cheaper. If you eat "safe starches," rice is also an option.

Canned fish such as wild-caught salmon can be a life-saver both in terms of convenience and economy. It was a boon for us Paleo types when it was discovered that farmed salmon didn't can well. Anchovies, tuna, herring, sardines, and the like can help to keep that protein cost per pound low.

Fresh deli fish like pre-cooked wild salmon that has been made ready to eat by prepping in lemon juice, water, and salt – can be even less expensive than canned tuna at $6 a pound.

Eat Out ONLY for Special Occasions

If you have children, many restaurants have certain nights that children eat free, which will make this luxury one that is a little less lavish. There are even smartphone apps that locate the kids' deals at restaurants, such as KidsEatFree.

Use the money you save to buy better quality foods for your health. The average cost increase of eating organic is 15% - 30% depending on location. You can look at it this way: Pay now or pay later in higher health care costs, not to mention the lower quality of life caused by health concerns. I am encouraged by the increased availability that I see now in organic foods, brought into existence, no doubt, by customers demanding it.

Visit Local Ethnic Markets for Bargains

For some substantial savings, try nationality stores in your area, where prices are often lower and variety better than in big box supermarkets, with special items you won't find there. For instance, check out your local Mexican meat market (carnicería) for goat meat (usually local and pastured) or mercado (traditional market) for other goods, Asian market (for veggies especially), or Indian market (usually half the price for the same brands of coconut milk). You need to be familiar with the usual prices in order to know what is a bargain, though, so do some research first. For instance, if you know that red peppers are $4.99 a pound at the big box grocery store, then you will take advantage when you see them for $1.50 a pound at the Asian grocery store.

Eat as Highly on the Health Spectrum as You Can

For each type of food, there are levels of healthiness among the different choices available in the marketplace. Of course, you would want to get the best that can be obtained within your means by eating as optimally as you can afford at the time.

Food	Good	Better	Best
Eggs	Normal	Free-Range	Cage-free
Fruits/Veg	Organic Frozen	Non-Organic Fresh	Organic Fresh
Meat	Organic Grain Fed	Organic Grass Fed	Organic Grass Fed and Finished
Oils	Organic Refined or Normal Unrefined	Organic Unrefined	Organic Virgin or Extra Virgin Unrefined

Paleo Compared to...

Let's get some perspective here. According to the USDA data, the average American spends $76 a week, $304 a month, on food. http://tinyurl.com/USDAdata Three meals a day at other less healthy alternatives don't come in so cheap, especially when you factor in the health consequences.

McDonald's Dollar Menu ... $270 a month

Paleo can run $30 a week if you use the tips in this book. Now, either quality or variety may have to suffer to come in this low, but it is totally doable. Here's an example that I saw on a blog:

You can do Monotonous Eating 101. 10 eggs for breakfast, prepared with pepper, onion powder, and salsa or hot sauce, scrambled, fried, however you like them (I'd add some veggies to that myself). You won't be hungry until dinner because of the huge protein load there, so you can get in some IF (intermittent fasting) doing that, too. At dinner, 16 ounces of 80/20 ground chuck sautéed with pepper, onion powder, chili powder, and hot sauce (Again, I'd add some veggies and/or fruit). The person doing this reported better mood, energy, and mental clarity, couple with weight loss to the tune of 21 pounds in 36 days with little to no exercise. Here's the break-down:

80/20 ground chuck, 6 lbs @ 2.78 a lb at Sam's Club

Eggs 7.5 dozen, 11.5 cents per egg at Sam's Club

Organic Unsalted Butter, x at Sam's Club

$4.22 per day, $29.54 per week, just $126.60 per month before you add in some less expensive veggies and fruits, about half of the Fast Food Dollar Menu comparison.

Optimal Paleo Eating

What are some of the factors to consider when buying Paleo foods? For example, I use a Google search for "Paleo [food name]" to find recipes for Paleo foods, but how do you know what is going to be in season at your local farmer's market? How do you know for sure which fats are healthy Paleo? What additives can be in non-organic foods? What about GMOs? What meats are best?

Seasonal Eating

Going further than just WHAT our ancestors ate, we can also consider WHEN they ate certain food sources, which was when that food was in its natural season. When that food was not available, it was not eaten. Today, everything is available everyday, but that was not how our species is designed to eat. To find your local produce in season, enter your state and the current season here: http://tinyurl.com/eatseasonal

Be sure to eat fat with your veggies! In summer, the most carbs can be eaten, but from October 15th to March 15th, eat only non-starchy veggies, with none at the winter solstice, to most closely follow ancestral eating habits.

Next, I'm including my personal research on the best fats, so that you can choose the healthiest to add to your veggies.

Lipids 101 – The Basics

"A false conclusion, once arrived at and widely accepted, is not dislodged easily, and the less it is understood, the more tenaciously it is held."

Cantor's Law of Preservation of Ignorance

http://tinyurl.com/heartsurgeonreveals

As a Paleo enthusiast, you probably already understand that all fats are not to be avoided and why, but just in case you are still worried about your hearth health, click the link above. Okay, so we can move on to which oils are best for you and which should be used with caution or in limited amounts, and which should be avoided.

So that you can more fully understand some of my recommendations later on, it is important for you to know the basics about fats and oils.

First, all fats and oils are made up of three kinds of fatty acids:

- Saturated

- Monounsaturated

- Polyunsaturated

The primary type of fatty acid contained in an oil will determine whether or not it should be exposed to oxygen, light, moisture, or heat. Those oils with large amounts of polyunsaturated fatty acids should never be used for cooking, only consumed raw, and only from raw, organic, cold-pressed, and unrefined sources. Oils with primarily polyunsaturated fatty acid components are easily damaged by heat, forming free radicals that cause inflammation, disease, and aging in the human body. For the same reasons, they should be stored in the refrigerator in an opaque, tightly sealed bottle.

Saturated fats are much more stable and resistant to damage from heat, so use them for cooking at higher temperatures – coconut oil, palm oil, butter, ghee, and lard. For sautéing at lower heat, you can safely use oils with high monounsaturated fatty acids and lower amounts of polyunsaturated fat, such as avocado oil, macadamia nut oil, and olive oil.

Since a saturated component has a protective effect on the oxidation of the polyunsaturated (and even monounsaturated) portion of the oil; when cooking, you can also add some saturated fat to any primarily monounsaturated fat for extra protection, although only some of them have significant polyunsaturated percentages, most notably peanut oil. sunflower oil, sesame oil, and rice bran oil, of which only sesame and rice bran oil can be added in small amounts, due to other issues with peanut and sunflower oils. Again, any oil with significant polyunsaturates should be cold-pressed, not refined, so that it has not been exposed to heat before you ever get it.

Trans fats are not a fat that exists in nature, but rather are manmade by hydrogenation of natural fats. They should never be eaten.

So how do we determine which fats and oils are best for us?

Several questions must be answered:

- What is the Omega-6 to Omega-3 ratio? We need this balance to be not more than 3:1 in our diet, preferably the 1:1 ratio on which our ancestors thrived. Today's typical ratios are closer to 20:1, much too high.

- Is the oil highly refined or not? Refining oils damages them.

- Is the oil hydrogenated or partially hydrogenated? Any oil that has been hydrogenated becomes a transfat, which is extremely unhealthy to eat.

- Does the oil come from a genetically modified organism (GMO)? GMO ingredients are not desirable.

- Are there antioxidants and/or vitamins in the oil? The more of these protective elements that are present, the more stable the oil.

Fats That Are Best to Eat

The list of good oils is much shorter, unfortunately, and usually much harder to find, especially in a grocery store.

Following are the good fats/oils I recommend:

- Extra Virgin Olive Oil (EVOO)

- Virgin Coconut Oil

- Udo's Choice Oil

- Avocado Oil

- Macadamia Nut Oil

- Organic Grass-Fed Butter

- Ghee

- Non-Hydrogenated Palm Oil

- Flax Seed Oil

- Fish Oil, Cod Liver Oil, or Krill Oil

- Lard

Extra Virgin Olive Oil (EVOO)

One of the oldest and safest oils, EVOO contains 75% oleic acid, the stable monounsaturated fat, along with 13% saturated fat, 10% omega-6 linoleic acid and 2% omega-3 linolenic acid. It is also rich in antioxidants, but don't overdo it. Long-chain fatty acids such as those found in olive oil are more likely to contribute to body fat than the short- and medium-chain fatty acids found in butter, coconut oil, or palm kernel oil. EVOO can be used for lower temperature cooking or as healthy salad dressing oil.

Virgin Coconut Oil

Maligned for years as a "bad" fat, coconut oil is very healthy when unrefined and unhydrogenated. Use only the virgin type. Virgin coconut oil contains medium chain triglycerides (MCTs) fatty acids, which are processed by the body differently from other oils, making them easier to digest because they are handled by the liver directly and can be used directly by the body as an energy source. In addition, they may benefit weight management because it can rev up your thyroid to stimulate the metabolism and give you energy. One study showed a significant reduction in waist circumference: http://tinyurl.com/VCOWaist

There's a somewhat humorous story about how farmers tried to use coconut oil in finishing feed to fatten cows, thinking that as a saturated fat, it would fatten them rapidly. This was a dismal failure, proving that coconut oil will not promote fat storage.

http://tinyurl.com/mctoil1

MCTs also affect gene expression away from adiposity: http://tinyurl.com/mctoil2

Another healthy advantage of this oil is its anti-viral, anti-fungal, and anti-bacterial properties, owing to its lauric acid content, which is also an immune system booster and a component of breast milk. It has super high stability under heat, making it ideal for all temperatures of cooking.

Udo's Choice Oil Blend

Udo's is a cold processed mechanically extracted blend of organic, non-GMO oils (coconut, sesame, sunflower, flax seed, evening primrose, rice bran, soy lecithin, oat germ and bran oil with mixed tocopherols) that mixes well with olive oil, garlic, vinegar, and onion to make salad dressings. It can be mixed into cottage cheese or protein shakes or other foods as well.

This blend must **never** be used for cooking, due to its higher polyunsaturated fat content, which means that heat would destroy the benefits of this oil. For the same reason, it must be kept refrigerated. Once opened, either use within 2 months or freeze to maintain freshness for longer periods. Udo's has a 2:1 Omega-6 to Omega-3 ratio, making it a healthy choice. Up to 1 tablespoon per 50 pounds body weight can be taken daily.

http://tinyurl.com/UdosChoiceOil

Avocado Oil

Relatively new on the market, cold pressed avocado oil has very low levels of acidity and oxidation products, but retains its vitamin E content. It can be used at high temperatures, up to 500 degrees, which is three times higher than that of olive oil. But, used in salads or salsa, it can significantly enhance the absorption of the carotenoids (lycopene, lutein, and beta-carotene), which are healthful antioxidants.

http://tinyurl.com/avocadooil1

If any of you watch Jamie Oliver's Food Revolution, he has stated in an interview in Elle magazine that avocado oil is the next "it" food ingredient in the culinary world. Avocado oil has been shown to be stable with regard to oxidation. http://tinyurl.com/avocadooil3

In some studies, the methods used must be called into question. For instance, this study comparing avocado oil, corn oil. coconut oil, and olive oil has a flaw in that the coconut oil and olive oils were not virgin (makes a huge difference). Not surprisingly, the coconut oil (not specified to be virgin and likely hydrogenated) had the worst atherogenicity. In addition, the avocado, coconut, and olive oils were not given alone, but rather had corn oil added, so the effects cannot be attributed solely to those oils, but likely is affected by the added corn oil. No wonder the other oils all came out to be similar in their effects to corn oil! Corn oil was added to those other oils, so what could you really expect? http://tinyurl.com/avocadooil4

Macadamia Nut Oil

This oil is one of the few with a perfect Omega-6 to Omega-3 balance of 1:1, but it has little of either, mostly Omega-9. Not only that, but it has very little polyunsaturated fat (4%) and mostly monounsaturated fat (83.5%), more than olive oil, most of it oleic acid, which facilitates the incorporation of Omega-3s into cell membranes. It does have 13% saturated fat, which somewhat protects the monounsaturated from damage when cooking, but should still be used at lower heats, not more than 410 degrees F. In a study testing the actual oxidative stability versus manufacturers' stated storage times, mac nut oil came in first in terms of its excellent resistance to rancidity.

http://tinyurl.com/macnutoil

Organic Grass-Fed Butter

Organic grass-fed butter supplies the healthy fatty acid CLA (conjugated linoleic acid), which can aid in burning fat and building muscle. Its Omega-6 to Omega-3 ratio is a better one than the usual commercial butters. KerryGold Irish butter is available at my local Costco. Sometimes I mix it up with some coconut oil and a touch of olive oil to use for cooking.

Ghee

Pure real ghee, which protects against free radicals and is resistant to free radical damage, is an ideal source of essential fatty acids. It is often called the supreme fat, so you may be surprised that you've never heard of it. It is clarified butter, something you may only be acquainted with in regard to a small container used for dipping lobster.

Traditional ghee is the essence of butter, without the lactose and other milk solids (good news for the lactose intolerant!). It is very easy to digest because it has 8% lower saturated fatty acids than any other edible oil. Ghee is made by cooking butter to caramelize the settled milk solids and then removing the solids to leave the pure fat. It is considered the supreme cooking oil because of its high flash (smoke) point, which allows it to be used at higher temperatures without damage, and its health-giving qualities, such as promoting digestion and elimination, making the complexion clear and bright.

Technically a saturated fat, ghee is different from other animal fats in that its molecular structure makes it a short-chain fatty acid (easily assimilated by the body) rather than a long-chain fatty acid (not metabolized by the body and leading to cancer and blood clots).

Although a saturated fat from animal origin, ghee is considered a vegetarian fat with many antioxidants such as Vitamin A and E to protect it from rancidity and oxidation, enabling it to remain fresh for three or four months when stored at room temperature out of the sun and away from moisture.

Non-Hydrogenated Palm Oil

You've probably been told that highly saturated fats like coconut and palm are unhealthy, and that's why they've been removed from the products in which they used to be found, such as coconut oil in crackers, pastries, and cookies, and clarified palm oil in shortening and commercial French fry oil. Unfortunately, they were replaced with hydrogenated oils such as soybean, corn, canola, and cottonseed. As you know, these ttrans fats are some of the worst for our health.

On the other hand, the very oils that were removed have been eaten by tropical populations for hundreds of years without causing heart disease. Palm oil is extremely stable for cooking and can be kept at room temperature for many months without becoming rancid. It has 300 times more carotenoid antioxidants than tomatoes, not to mention the Vitamin E antioxidants present, so it is both safe and healthy, contrary to what you might have heard. The domestic vegetable oil industry lobbied strongly to influence this change through the saturated fat scare. And our health has been the worse for it.

Several clinical studies show the benefits of this healthy oil:

http://tinyurl.com/palmoil1
http://tinyurl.com/palmoil2
http://tinyurl.com/palmoil3

Flax Seed Oil

While not suitable for cooking, flax seed oil is a good way to balance out your Omega-3/Omega-6 ratio by getting more Omega-3, not found abundantly in other oils. Flax seed oil has over 50% Omega-3 to use making salad dressing or spread.

Another plant-based Omega-3 source is chia seeds, freshly ground at the time of consumption, or soaked in water for 10 minutes to form a gel. The advantage of flax or chia is that they are vegan sources of Omega-3 fatty acids. However, when compared to fish-based forms, the Omega-3 in flax and chia is ALA (alpha linolenic acid), while the omega-3 fats in fish oil, cod liver oil and krill oil are DHA (docosahexaenoic acid) and EPA (eicosapentaenoic acid), which are considered to be superior in that most of the benefits of Omega-3 are associated with DHA rather than ALA. http://tinyurl.com/fishoilvsflax

Caution: Too much flax oil may trigger mania in about half of the bi-polar population.

Fish Oil, Cod Liver Oil, or Krill Oil

Fish oil is preferred over flax if you are only going to take one. In winter months, fish oil will also supply needed Vitamin D that flax will not. Consuming both is a good idea for balance.

Because fish oil can be contaminated with toxins, however, you might want to test yours by puncturing them with a needle and squeezing the oil into a small thimble, shotglass, or similar container. After freezing for 5 hours, if a toothpick can be easily pushed into the oil, it is less likely that there would be significant contamination.

http://tinyurl.com/fishoil2
http://tinyurl.com/fishoil3

Caution: Too much fish oil may trigger mania in about half of the bi-polar population.

Lard

Real lard is rendered pork fat that is naturally-hydrogenated, solid fat. It is not the lard found in tubs or boxes on grocery shelves, but rather should be stored in the refrigerator case.

In 1909, shortening was a natural product made with coconut oil and lard. Shortening used today is made out of partially hydrogenated vegetable oil. Why has lard been demonized as the worst kind of fat?

Comparing lard to human breast milk fat content, saturated fat is similar (48% in human milk, 42% in lard), monounsaturated has the most variance (35% in human milk, 44% in lard), and polyunsaturated is exactly the same, 10%.(Rounding makes the numbers not add up to 100%.)

How does lard stack up against olive oil, which almost everyone agrees is healthy? Olive oil contains 71% oleic acid versus 44% oleic acid in lard, which is more than is found in beef tallow (43%), butterfat (29%), and human breast milk at 35%.

Other fatty acids are similar, except for palmitic acid, which lard contains twice as much of as olive oil (26% vs 13%). In comparison, human breast milk contains 25%, almost exactly the same, so how could the amount in lard be excessive?

I never heard of some of these oils. Where do I find them?

Some of these healthy oils must be found online or in health food stores, but a very few are available in regular groceries.

Fats to Use in Limited Amounts

These oils can be used in limited amounts, due to the high Omega-6 content:

- Sesame oil
- Rice bran oil

Sesame Oil

Sesame oil has 43% Omega-6 fatty acids, but it also has unique antioxidants that that are not destroyed by heat. It is flavorful, especially when toasted, and could be used in small amounts for added flavor.

Rice Bran Oil

Rice bran oil shows some benefits in many areas of health, including suppressing hyperinsulinemic responses and improving insulin sensitivity in diabetics.

http://tinyurl.com/RiceBOil1   http://tinyurl.com/RiceBOil2
http://tinyurl.com/RiceBOil3

However, contaminants such as pesticides have been reported in rice bran oil used for cooking. Moreover, it has some of the same concerns as some of the other oils, hexane used in refining and too much Omega-6 fatty acid (33%). Compared to olive oil, rice bran oil has four times more Omega-6. Unless you can find cold-pressed rice bran oil (NOT cold-filtered, which is marketing meant to confuse you into thinking it is cold-pressed), it should not be used, and even then, I'd limit the use due to the high Omega-6.

Fats to Avoid Altogether

In order of worst to least worst:

- Trans fats of all kinds, which are hydrogenated oils or partially hydrogenated oils. Even a healthy oil that has been hydrogenated now becomes an unhealthy one.

- Canola Oil

- Soybean Oil

- Corn Oil

- Safflower Oil

- Peanut Oil

- Cottonseed Oil

- Grape Seed Oil

- Sunflower Oil

Even if you are not buying oil, you still need to consider whether the ingredients of any products contain the oils to avoid. Consider that nearly all store-bought salad dressings (and even mayo) contain soybean oil, even those that might claim olive oil as an ingredient on the front of the label. When you read the back of the label, you discover that the bulk of the oil in the product is soybean or canola.

Trans fats

I remember reading about nutrition back in the late 70's, when people were encouraged to substitute margarine for butter,

73

because people thought that the margarine was more healthy because it didn't have saturated fats and cholesterol, which were just starting to be demonized at that time as causing heart disease. Even back then, some nutritionists knew the truth that margarine was LESS healthy than butter due to the hydrogenated oils (ttrans fats), and were already sounding the alarm. This resulted in my never having switched to margarine, and I'm so glad that I knew better from doing research.

And look how many decades it took for the mainstream to catch up to understanding that margarine with ttrans fats was an unhealthy choice. It's very difficult for those who have loudly proclaimed something to admit that they were wrong, wrong, WRONG. That's why it's taking so long for it to be accepted that all saturated fats are not bad for you.

Be sure to check the labels of any standard processed products before you buy, because you will be shocked to see that you will find hydrogenated oils (ttrans fats). These can hide in such products as mainstream peanut butter, for heaven's sake. Most natural type peanut butter has none, but I would limit even that as well, due to several studies linking peanut oil to fibrous lesions on the arteries, which is explained later in this chapter.

Canola Oil

Contrary to what you may have been told, canola oil is not heart healthy at all. The processing of canola oil and oxidation of the polyunsaturated component of canola oil makes it unhealthy and inflammatory in your body.

Although you've been told by the mainstream media that canola oil is a healthy source of monounsaturated fats similar to olive oil, nothing could be further from the truth. In the case of virgin olive oil, its monounsaturated fats are healthy for you, because the oil is not highly processed using heat and solvents to enhance the extraction process the way that canola and other processed and refined oils are. Extra virgin olive oil has other protective properties such as antioxidants.

Even though canola oil is high in monounsaturates (55-65%), it also contains polyunsaturates (28-35%), which are damaged by heavy processing such as that undergone by canola oil, soybean oil, and corn oil. These highly processed and refined vegetable oils have polyunsaturates that are damaged by those refining methods, since they are highly unstable under heat, light, and pressure, not to mention the caustic and questionable chemicals such as hexane, a petroleum solvent used in the refining process.

All of these methods transform some of the Omega-3 fatty acids into harmful ttrans fats and oxidize the polyunsaturates, increasing free radicals in your body when you ingest it. Ultimately, the oil increases inflammation in the body, which can potentially contribute to degenerative diseases such as heart disease and weight gain.

If all of this information doesn't convince you, then watch the video comparisons of the process to make butter versus the process to make canola oil: http://tinyurl.com/buttervscanola Unless the canola oil that you find is organic and cold-pressed, it will be the highly processed kind just described, something to avoid. This would apply to any of the "avoid" oils, but even cold-pressed, many of these, such as safflower, corn, sunflower, soybean and cottonseed oils, all contain over 50% omega-6 and, except for soybean oil, only minimal amounts of omega-3.

This is a problem because unlike omega-3 fatty acids, omega-6 has serious side effects if ingested in excess. According to The Ohio State University Research News, if omega-6 and omega-3 are in a one-to-one proportion to each other in the diet, this does not happen, because they balance each other out. The American diet is already highly skewed towards Omega-6, unfortunately, which has been shown to contribute to depression and inflammatory diseases. More Omega-6 in your diet is not what you are looking for when you want good health. http://tinyurl.com/omega3omega6

Soybean Oil

Everything said about canola oil also applies to soybean oil, and in addition, over 90% of the soybeans available in the United States are genetically modified organisms (GMO) which other countries have banned, and rightfully so. Furthermore, since most Americans are out of balance with respect to Omega-3 fatty acids and Omega-6 fatty acids, which should be in the diet in equal amounts for optimum health, soybean oil has so much more Omega-6 fatty acids than Omega-3 that it only makes this worse.

Corn Oil

Another highly refined oil with inflammatory properties, corn oil also bears the same onus as soybean oil, in that over 90% of the corn in the United States is GMO.

This oil can be especially dangerous to consume, given that it has been seen in a clinical study to have epigenetic effects to change genetic expression to activate genes associated with prostate cancer development. The Omega-6 fatty acid arachidonic acid is the culprit: http://tinyurl.com/cornoilcancer

Safflower Oil

Safflower oil contains almost 80% omega-6 fatty acid content, not a good choice at all. Even if you find an unrefined version, cooking with this oil will damage it. Eating it will further skew your Omega-6 to Omega-3 balance to an unhealthy ratio.

Sunflower Oil

Sunflower oil is another oil typically refined, and containing 35% Omega-6 fatty acids. Only an unrefined cold-pressed version such as that in Udo's Blend is acceptable for use, and don't forget that cooking with this oil will damage it.

Peanut Oil

Peanut oil has 34% Omega-6 fatty acids, but is fairly stable in terms of oxidation and would be suitable for occasional use, were it not for the fact that it has no Omega-3 at all, and these studies, which show that it can promote lesions on arterial walls, apparently associated with the biologically active lectin that it contains, which has a specific affinity for the glycoproteins on the arterial walls:

http://tinyurl.com/peanutoil   http://tinyurl.com/peanutoil2
http://tinyurl.com/peanutoil3 http://tinyurl.com/peanutoil4

Grape Seed Oil

Grape seed oil contains 71% polyunsaturated fats and should never be exposed to any degree of heat. Contamination with mineral oil paraffin has been reported: http://tinyurl.com/gsoil It is also typically refined, so if you do use it, only cold-pressed unrefined is acceptable.

Cottonseed Oil

Often genetically modified, usually hydrogenated to form a transfat, and almost always refined, cottonseed oil is not one recommended to use. The original Crisco that replaced the animal fat based shortening that had been formerly used for baking was cottonseed oil based, hence the name: CRYStalized Cottonseed Oil.

Organic Food Free from Additives

I know what you are thinking. "I thought that you said that we don't have to eat organic, in order to eat Paleo." You don't. It is closer to what our ancestors ate, since they didn't have the toxic pesticides used today, so I do think that you want to be educated about why organic would be a good investment if you can shift some expenses around to accommodate it in your spending plan. If you know that you can't or won't, you can just skip this section. I still believe that eating Paleo without eating organic is a much better choice than sticking with the SAD way of eating that most folks still embrace, to the detriment of their long-term (and sometimes short-term) health and well-being.

Ironically, the initial movement towards increasing crop/livestock yields using pesticides, herbicides, fungicides, synthetic fertilizers, genetically engineered organisms (GMOs), routine antibiotics for otherwise healthy animals, and hormones such as rGBH or rBST in raising livestock and produce, was called the Green Revolution. Yep, not exactly what we think of as "green" today, which is currently used to denote a good thing for our environment.

Here's what you need to know to shop smart for healthy food.

What does organic mean?

100% organic, that's the best. The next is probably certified organic, then organic and last would be made with organic, which means next to nothing.

How can I tell if produce is organic?

9=organic; Add a '9' in front of the four digit PLU code. An organically grown standard yellow banana would be '94011'.

8=GE; Add an '8' in front of the four digit PLU code. A genetically engineered standard yellow banana would be '84011'. www.PLUcodes.com http://tinyurl.com/PLUguide

What is a GMO?

A genetically modified organism (GMO) is a plant, animal or microorganism whose genetic code has been altered (subtracted from, or added to either the same species or a different species) in order to give it characteristics that it does not have naturally.

Scientists can now transfer genes between species that otherwise would be incapable of mating, for example, a goat and a spider. This is what we call transgenesis. Little is known about the long-term effects of such manipulations on humans, plants, animals and/or the environment. And while some see GMOs as the way to the future, others believe that scientists have gone too far, tinkering with the essence of life.

What's the difference between "all natural" and "organic"?

All natural refers to no additives and *is based on testimony of the producer*. **Organic** means the product comes from at least 90% organic ingredients, but **100% organic** means 100% of the ingredients are organic. **Certified organic** must come from animals whose parents were certified raised organic and raised from birth on organic land. They must be fed organic crops. The land cannot have been sprayed with pesticides, herbicides, fungicides, or synthetic fertilizers for a minimum of 3 years prior to certification. No animal byproducts may be fed to certified organic animals. No genetically engineered organisms (GMOs) may be used in feed or the animals. The product to be certified must be documented from birth to purchaser for traceability and verification. Antibiotics cannot be used in organic meat.

What's the difference between the different types of meat?

o **Regular beef** is usually kept very contained and fed hormones, antibiotics and supplements as well as grains, and ground-up animal by-products. Most of the animal by-products are from animals that were sick and not fit for human consumption. (Cows are not supposed to eat meat!!) Since the animals are contained, they don't get any exercise and toxins aren't able to be released from their bodies.

o Some animals are given all the hormones, antibiotics, and supplements as well as the grains and animal by-products but allowed time to roam free. In my area this is called **free-range meat**.

o **All natural beef** starts its life as regular beef but is allowed to roam free in the fields and is not given any hormones, antibiotics, or supplements for at least the last few months of its life. It is still fed grains. It's better than regular beef.

o **Organic beef** is never given any hormones, antibiotics, supplements, etc. Neither have their parents. They are never given any feed that is grown with the use of pesticides or chemical fertilizers. (The ground can't have been sprayed for at least 3 years where the feed is grown.) The animals are treated by natural methods if they become ill. If that doesn't work and the farmer needs to use an injection to cure the animal, it is labeled and sold as regular beef. These animals are free to roam their entire lives. They are also fed grains.

o **Grass fed only organic beef** is never fed grains. They eat in the fields and are fed hay when weather doesn't permit them to free graze. The proven benefits of eating "Grass-Only Beef" include: less fat, fewer calories, more Omega-3 fatty acids, a healthier ratio of Omega-6 to Omega-3 fatty acids, more Conjugated Linoleic Acid (CLA), more Vitamin E, and higher levels of beta-carotene. This is the best meat.

Found Money – Expense Category-Shifting Ideas

Chapter 3

In the US, we spend less on food at the grocery store, per capita as a percentage of gross income, than almost any other country – 9%. And that's a real shame, in that it tends to show that we don't value the quality of food we consume, despite how deeply it influences the state of our health. We spend less than most industrialized nations with higher incomes, so it's not just because we make more money than some other country's citizens.

By contrast, 111 years ago, the average American spent almost half of their income on food, according to the Bureau of Labor Statistics. Only 3% of that was spent on eating out, compared to closer to half of the food expense in America going to food outside the home now.

About 63 years ago, 22% was the average expense for food as a portion of income in America. Factory farming methods have brought food prices way down, arguably teaching us to expect food to be cheap, but at what cost? Your health. We now spend much less on food, but correspondingly much more on medical bills and prescriptions. Those numbers aren't unrelated.

Americans used to be willing to spend more on food that was of higher quality. And we were much healthier then. We have to place a higher priority on healthy food, not cheap food. We can do this in a smart way, using the information in this book to save money while still getting the most healthy food sources that we can afford.

However, we can also shift our priorities, consciously taking some money from other expense categories in order to use it to improve the quality of the food we buy. After all, haven't you heard the saying that you can pay the farmer (or grocer) or you can pay the doctor?

If you need even one less prescription, think of the savings from that per month. Co-pays have gone way up, so even if you have insurance, it is a significant expense. Medical bills from becoming ill more often are also costly. Someone I respect greatly, Dr Jack Kruse, wrote on his blog recently, "Cheap food leads to expensive medicine." Unless you know the secrets for getting healthy food less expensively, like those given in this book, that is certainly the case.

Saving money in other areas of your life means more is available for healthy Paleo food. Very few people realize the many opportunities that abound for saving money with little effort. By taking advantage of these tips, you can use the savings to improve your health, which in the end will also save you money on doctor's bills, prescriptions, and co-pays.

Gasoline Savings

You can save from 10 to 50% on gasoline every month! Here are ideas to save on one of our most expensive costs these days:

- Monitor your tire pressure and keep them properly inflated to save an additional 2% on your mileage.

- Don't postpone vehicle maintenance. It pays for itself in improved mileage, not to mention fewer repairs or tows that you might need if you delay. Tune-ups and other vehicle maintenance can give you 4 to 40% better mileage.

- Just changing your air filter can improve your mileage by 10%

- Join a carpool or just agree to share rides a couple of times a week with a nearby coworker or neighbor.

- Ask if you can work from home at least once a week.

- For even more savings, consider starting a home-based business that can eventually replace your present job.

82

Utility Savings

I might be the only person in America not to have known this fact, but I was shocked to learn that many appliances are using electricity even when they are not turned on, if they are still plugged in. Who knew? Not me. There is even a name for it-- vampire power. It is caused by the power drain of what is called "auxiliary power or "aux power" that allows appliances to turn on faster when you press the power button on, to run a timer, or to turn on by use of a remote control. Estimates of the percentage of annual power consumption can be 5-20%.

Cordless appliances with rechargeable batteries are notorious for sucking more electricity when "off" but still plugged in, even when the battery is fully charged. Corded appliances are much less likely to use significant power when off and still attached to power sources. Larger power adapters and those that feel warm to the touch are more prone to use more than one watt of power when off.

If you want to know what it costs to leave an appliance plugged in while it's not being used, you can get a little gadget called a Kill A Watt for under $20: http://tinyurl.com/killingwatts It can even help you to decide whether it is more cost effective to keep an older appliance that uses more power, or to replace it with a newer one that consumes less power, even in standby mode. But if it isn't possible to consider replacing older appliances, don't despair of being able to decrease this expense.

Ever since I have identified the appliances that don't have to be on all the time (such as toasters, coffee makers, blenders, food processors, computers, lamps, fans, hairdryers, flat irons, and so on), and plugged them all into power strips rather than directly into the wall socket, it has allowed me to **really** turn something off when I don't need it. I just flip the switch "off" on the power strip, instead of using the one on the appliance itself. My utility bill has noticeably reduced from this one tip.

Online Discount Resources

Use online resources to find out what's on sale, or what coupons could give you a discount.

National Discount Sites

<u>Groupon</u>: Offers Daily Deals on everything. Average discount: 50%.

<u>LivingSocial</u>: Another large Daily Deal site, with a twist that can save you money. You get the deal you purchased FREE after you share it with three friends who also buy the same deal. It's called Me+3.

<u>Angie's List</u>: Through Angie's The Big Deal program, you can get discount offers on home services ranging from A/C inspection to maid services.

<u>Scoutmob</u>: Phone app or email signups give you daily deals for restaurants and personal services, as well as reviews of local events and vendors in larger cities

Aggregator Discount Sites

<u>Google Offers</u>: Based on your location, gives you discount offers for local businesses.

<u>8coupons</u>: Shows you the deals closest to you.

Social Media Discounts and Coupons

<u>Facebook</u>: Use the search tool to see if a favorite product or company offers daily email deals.

<u>Twitter</u>: Follow <u>@EarlyBird</u>, <u>@CheapTweet</u>, <u>@CouponTweet</u>

Miscellaneous Savings Tips

Keep your thermostat 1 degree chillier to save 1-2% in winter.

Get your books from the library instead of buying them. If you need a copy to keep, try Goodwill or Half Price Books, where books can often be found on clearance for $1.00 Don't forget that Half Price Books sends you additional savings in coupons if you sign up for their mailing list or email list.

Go to matinee movies instead of full-price. Be sure to ask for any discounts for which you qualify, such as student or senior citizen ticket prices. I got a kick out of the irony of buying a senior citizen ticket for the first time for the Hunger Games, a movie based on a young adult novel I enjoyed.

Barter with people for things you need. This can work even at garage sales, if a bigger ticket item is out of your price range; but you have a skill or another item that the owner would like.

Bring dinner leftovers to work for lunch, and save the expense of eating out every day for lunch, a practice that can potentially save $100 per month all by itself.

Think about what you can get rid of in your life. Surely something is unnecessary, or at least not as critical to your health as your food really is. Maybe you can drive a car that is not as fancy, or eliminate part of your cable or satellite TV bill by not having all the premium channels. Evaluate what is really important to you and make adjustments accordingly.

Found Time – Make Your Own Convenience Foods

Chapter 4

What I have noticed is that the times that I did not eat Paleo as I'd intended to do are also the times that I did not plan ahead to make it easy and convenient for me to do. Or I ate out because I wasn't prepared with food that was easy to get ready at home. Here are some ways to pre-prepare Paleo "convenience foods" so that you always have something that can be ready in minutes instead of hours.

Lots of money goes down the drain in processed or prepared foods. DIY can save you lots of money and is almost always healthier because you know what you used as ingredients. As an example, broth or stock bought in a store often has MSG or other additives, even sugar. If you make your own bone broth, you know what it contains. Ghee can be made at home, and so can many other Paleo staples, such as salad dressings, mayo, jerky, salsa, almond meal and flour, kefir and sauerkraut and pickles, bone broth or stock, lard, suet, butter, yogurt, canned veggies, dried fruit, sauces and marinades, meatza, and, believe it or not, paleo-type crackers, chips, breads, muffins, pancakes and waffles, coffee creamer, desserts, and cakes.

Recipe Abbreviations:

T = Tablespoon

t = teaspoon

C = Cup

Basics

Bone Broth

Bone broth is incredibly healthy for you, but do be sure to use bones from grass-fed, clean animals (not given hormones or antibiotics). Save all bones, meat scraps, and veggie scraps in a zippered plastic bag in the freezer. When it's full, empty it into your crock pot with 4 quarts of water and 1-2 tsp. of vinegar to help pull the nutrients and gelatin and marrow from the bones. Some folks like to roast the bones first in a 400-degree oven, to give an even richer flavor. You can add smashed garlic cloves, celery, onion, or any other spices you like. Turn it on the high setting to get to a boil, then down to low heat for 24-36 hours. Or use your pressure cooker to get 'er done in less than an hour.

Strain the result and freeze in ice trays or silicone cupcake pans. When frozen, you can transfer to zippered freezer bags for convenient individual servings to use as a drink or in soups, chilis, stews, sauces, and other dishes.

Beef, pork, lamb, chicken, turkey, or other birds, all types of bones can be used to make bone broth. Game meats can also be used to make great bone broth or stock. Your butcher can sell you bones dirt-cheap if you don't have leftover bones from bone-in cuts of meat you bought. You'll get hooked on this quickly, and even might start pestering others to save their bones for you, if they don't save them for themselves.

Bone broth gives you many minerals that you might be lacking if you do not eat dairy on your type of Paleo. Gelatin, collagen, chondroitin sulfates, and glucosamine provide health-giving benefits, too. The collagen is even said to improve the appearance of cellulite due to the connective tissue repair. When your bone broth is cold, you can tell whether the nutrients have been extracted from the bones well, by how gelatinous it is, which is what you want for good rich stock.

Sauces

Meat Sauce

Bone Broth
1/2 t Rosemary
1/2 t Sage
1/4 t Savory (optional)

2 cloves Garlic, minced
1/3 small fresh jalapeno pepper or red chili, chopped finely

You can leave out the pepper if you don't like a spicy sauce. Or you can adjust the amount after chopping the whole pepper. I would wait 10 minutes or so before tasting, to let the flavors develop. After reducing, add a T of coconut milk at a time if you like.

Another sumptuous meat sauce is this one:

Meat Sauce 2

4 T butter, divided
1/4 C Onion, chopped
1/4 C Garlic, chopped
1/2 C Lemon juice
Bone Broth
1/2 C White Wine
Kosher Salt to taste
White Pepper to taste

Sauté 1 Tbsp. butter, onions and garlic. Add juice, broth, and wine. Simmer at medium-low heat until reduced by 90%. Cool slightly and gradually add remaining butter, stirring constantly, until it emulsifies, but not so hot that it separates.

Frozen Sautéed Mushrooms for Sauces

2 pounds Mushrooms, sliced (any variety)
1/2 C Extra Virgin Coconut Oil
4 Green Onions, finely chopped
1/3 C White Wine (optional)
4 T Butter or Ghee
6 cloves Garlic, minced
2 t Kosher Salt
1/2 t Pepper

Sauté green onions in coconut oil on medium-high. Add the mushrooms and butter or ghee. Sauté for a few minutes. Add the white wine after the butter has melted, add in the white wine and deglaze for about 5 minutes to let the mushrooms absorb the wine. Next, add the garlic and simmer two minutes. Let cool for 1/2 hour. Place in zippered bags for the freezer.

Want to thicken a sauce without flour or cornstarch? Coconut cream concentrate is the secret to this one. By mixing a tablespoon of coconut cream with half a cup of hot water, you can then whisk that into anything you are trying to thicken. This is great if you are avoiding dairy, because you can make a creamy tomato soup with this method, sans butter or cream. Other Paleo-friendly thickeners would be arrowroot, coconut milk, xanthan gum, guar gum, or ThickNot.

Salad Dressings

The Salad Dressing Matrix

Dressings are really just a mix of three basic ingredients: Oil, Acid, and Herbs. So we can make a matrix of the choices available from those three ingredients and come up with a "Chose one from Column A and one from Column B and then one or more from Column C" as the easy-peasy dressing choices matrix.

Now, yes, some combos will be better than others, because some things just naturally taste better together, but in general, this is just not that complicated. Add 3 parts of oil with each 1 part of acid and herbs to taste.

Mix the herbs (especially salt, which needs to dissolve thoroughly) with the acid first. Then add the oil by drizzling it very slowly while simultaneously whisking enthusiastically. Remember, you can use a blender or a food processor to avoid repetitive stress injury from whisking manually. Keep in mind that if you choose Dijon mustard as one of your herbs, it fosters the emulsion of oil with acid, as well as adding a tang.

Acids – 1 Part	Herbs – to Taste	Oils – 3 Parts
Apple Cider Vinegar	Green Onions	Extra Virgin Olive Oil
Balsamic Vinegar	Cilantro	Coconut Oil
Rice Vinegar	Thyme	Avocado Oil
Red Wine Vinegar	Turmeric	Macadamia Oil
Lemon Juice	Coriander	Sesame Oil (dash for flavor)
Lime Juice	Cinnamon	Rice Bran Oil (dash for flavor)
Tomato Juice	Paprika	Mayonnaise
	Smoked Paprika	Greek Yogurt
	Ginger	Yogurt
	Cayenne	Buttermilk
	Cumin	Plain Kefir
	Garlic	Sour Cream
	Basil	Cottage Cheese
	Oregano	
	Chili Pepper	
	Chipotle	
	Red Pepper Flakes	
	White, Yellow, Or Red Onions	
	Dill	
	Black Pepper	
	Mint	
	Mustard	
	Anchovy Paste	
	Tamari	
	Honey	
	Nuts	
	Cheeses	

Dressings created with the Matrix can also be used for marinades, but not for more than an hour if using acids. If you consume it on your version of Paleo, you can use dairy with some acidic component to it (sour cream, Greek yogurt, buttermilk, or kefir) in your dressings, too. Dairy can be left for longer than more acidic marinades.

Ranch Dressing

3/4 C Mayonnaise
1/4 C Buttermilk
1/2 t Garlic Powder
Dash of Minced Garlic
1/4 t Cayenne Pepper
1/4 t Fresh Cracked Black Pepper

Basic Dressing

1/4 C Apple Cider Vinegar
3/4 C Extra Virgin Olive Oil
3 T Bragg's Amino Acids
1/4 t White Pepper
1/4 t Cayenne Pepper
Stevia to taste

Another Basic Dressing

1/4 C Balsamic Vinegar
3/4 C Coconut Oil
2 cloves Garlic, minced finely
1/4 t Oregano
1/4 t Basil
Stevia to taste

Yet Another Basic Dressing

1/4 C Rice Vinegar
3/4 C Extra Virgin Olive Oil
2 cloves Garlic, minced finely
2 T Dijon Mustard
2 or 3 Green Onions, finely chopped
Freshly Ground Black Pepper
Sea Salt

Onion Salad Dressing

1 T Chopped Onion
1/4 Lemon, juiced

1/4 t Basil
1/4 t Oregano
1/4 t Cumin
Sea Salt
Freshly Ground Black Pepper

Dressing for Raw Veggies

1/2 T Dill Weed
1 1/2 T Apple Cider Vinegar
4 1/2 T Avocado Oil
Stevia to taste (optional)

Sprinkle fresh dill on any veggie after marinating lightly in apple cider vinegar and avocado oil. If needed, add a little stevia. This really brings out the natural flavors.

Dressing for Raw Cucumbers

1/4 C Apple Cider Vinegar
1/4 C Bragg's Amino Acids
Stevia to taste

Marinade for Steak, Fish, and Chicken

3/4 C Coconut Oil
1/4 C Coconut Milk
1/2 Lemon, juiced
1/2 t Ginger, minced finely
2 cloves Garlic, minced finely

Amazon has some jarred Homemade Dressing Mixes that I just love, and they are eligible for Subscribe and Save, too!
http://tinyurl.com/HomemadeDressings

Condiments

Homemade Mayonnaise

2 large Egg Yolks
3 T Lemon Juice
1/4 t Sea Salt

Pinch of White Pepper
1 C Extra Light Olive Oil

Put the yolks, lemon juice, salt, and pepper into a mixing bowl and whisk until smooth and light. Then whisk the oil, a few drops at a time, into the mixture. Ensure the mixture is smooth and well integrated before pouring the next few drops of oil.

The whisking will suspend the oil into the yolk mixture and adding the oil a little at a time will keep the mixture in a state of emulsion. After about 1/3 C of the oil has been whisked in, you can speed up the pouring a bit. Ensure the mixture is back in emulsion before pouring any more oil. After all the oil has been whisked in, you have mayonnaise. You can also use your blender or food processor to avoid repetitive stress injury.

Because homemade mayonnaise is mostly egg yolk, the mayonnaise will have a healthy yellow color. Refrigerate in a tightly sealed jar and it should stay fresh for a week.

Variations:

Use some liquid bacon fat in place of some or all of the oil. Use coconut oil for up to half of the oil.

Homemade Mustard

Avoid the sugar and other additives we don't need by making your mustard from scratch.

1/2 C White Wine Vinegar
1/2 C Dry Mustard Powder
1/4 t Ground Allspice
1 t Turmeric
1 t Sea Salt

Place all ingredients in a food processor and process until smooth. Add cold water if consistency is too thick. Refrigerate in airtight container for at least 12 hours and up to two weeks before serving.

Variations: Add some horseradish or chipotle for a spicy tang!

Homemade Honey Mustard

2 C Homemade Mayonnaise
2/3 C Homemade Mustard
1 T Raw Honey
4 T Lemon Juice

Mix all ingredients thoroughly and store refrigerated in an airtight container.

Homemade Cocktail Sauce

1 C Sugar-Free Tomato Sauce
1 T Onion, minced
1/2 T Celery Salt
1/4 T Paprika
2 T Fresh Chopped Parsley
1 T Stevia
1 T Worcestershire Sauce
1 T Fresh Lemon Juice
2 T Drained, Prepared Horseradish
1/2 t Hot Sauce
Cumin to taste
Sea Salt to taste
Freshly Ground Black Pepper to taste

Homemade Mexican Cocktail Sauce

1 C Fresh Salsa
1/2 C Sugar Free Tomato Juice
2 T Onion, minced
1/2 t Cilantro
1/2 T Lemon or Lime Juice

Use cayenne or Tabasco and add a little Stevia if you don't like it tart.

Homemade Tzatziki Sauce

8 oz. Plain Yogurt, drained
3 T Extra Virgin Olive Oil

1 t Dill
1 Medium Cucumber
4 cloves Garlic, minced
Sea Salt to taste
Freshly Ground Black Pepper to taste

Shred a cucumber, put it in a paper towel, and press out the water. Mix everything and you have the best Tzatziki. Refrigerate for at least 1 hour to let the tastes meld. If you really want to make true Tzatziki, buy Greek yogurt. A good brand is Total or Greek Gods brands of yogurt. There is no comparison between full fat Greek yogurt and drained American yogurt.

Homemade Sugar-Free Catsup

Boil several tomatoes for 10 minutes, or use a can of organic sugar-free tomato paste plus 1/3 C water. Put in food processor with a bit of garlic, a pinch each of cloves and allspice, 1/4 t each of cinnamon and dry mustard, 2 T either vinegar or lemon juice, and 1/4 t sea salt. Keep in the refrigerator. Add a pinch of Stevia if you want a sweeter flavor and a pinch of cayenne if you like it spicy.

Homemade BBQ Sauce

1 t Liquid Smoke or 1 t Smoked Paprika or Chipotle Powder
1 Small Onion, Minced
1 Clove Garlic, Minced or 1/4 t Garlic Powder
1 Small Can Sugar-Free (6 Oz) Tomato Paste
Stevia to taste
1/4 C Sugar-Free Catsup
3 T Mustard
1 T Worcestershire Sauce
Pinch of Ground Cloves
Hot Sauce to taste
1/2 C of Water

Pan-fry the onion in the Liquid Smoke over medium flame for about 4 minutes. Add garlic clove and stir. Add the remaining ingredients, including the water. Stir. Allow to simmer for 20-30 minutes. Stevia will tone down the spiciness if needed.

Variation: Add 1/2 C Apple Cider Vinegar to make it tangier.

Homemade Worcestershire Sauce

1/2 C Apple Cider Vinegar
2 T Water
2 T Soy Sauce or Wheat-Free Tamari
1/4 t Ground Ginger
1/4 t Mustard Powder
1/4 t Onion Powder
1/4 t Garlic Powder
1/8 t Cinnamon
1/8 t Freshly Ground Black Pepper

Bring all ingredients to a boil, constantly stirring. Simmer for a minute or two. Cool and refrigerate.

Homemade Salsa

1 T Water
1/2 small Tomato
2 slices Onion
1/4 t Oregano
1/4 t Chili Pepper
1/4 t Red Pepper
1/4 t Minced Garlic
Sea Salt to taste
Freshly Ground Black Pepper to taste

Blend in food processor/blender with small amount of water.

Homemade Salsa, Too

2 medium Tomatoes, diced or chopped
1/4 t Cilantro
1/4 t Cayenne
1/4 Lemon, juiced

2 t Apple Cider Vinegar
Sea Salt to taste

Blend the tomatoes and add spices.

Homemade Green Salsa

2 medium Green Tomatoes
1/4 t Minced Garlic
1/4 t Cilantro
Water to desired consistency
Sea Salt to taste

Blanch tomatoes and peel off skin. Boil until tender. Use
food processor or blender to mix.

Seasoning Mixes

Homemade Taco Seasoning for Taco Salad

2 t Paprika
1 1/2 t Sea Salt
1 t Onion Powder
1 t Chili Powder
1 1/2 t Cumin
1/2 t Garlic Powder

For more kick, add a pinch of cayenne pepper.

Blackened Chicken Seasoning

2 t Paprika
1 t Onion Powder
1 t Garlic Powder
1/4 t Cayenne Pepper
1/2 t White Pepper
1/2 t Black Pepper
1/2 t Sea Salt
1/2 t Thyme
1/2 t Oregano

Miscellaneous Convenience Foods

Homemade Beef Jerky

Store-bought jerky inevitably has brown sugar in it, if not other things you don't want to eat, such as nitrates and preservatives. Making your own is the perfect solution to this problem. For instance, beef cuts might be flank steak, top round steak, and rump roast .Beef, bison, chicken, ostrich, pork, salmon, turkey, and venison can all be made into jerky.

If you cut the meat yourself, remember to cut against the grain and to put the meat in the freezer for a bit first to make it easier to cut. You can always ask the butcher to cut it for you, though. Strips of 1/4 inch wide work well.

To season your jerky, of course, YOU will leave out the brown sugar that commercial manufacturers use. Here's a marinade mixture that works well:

2 T cloves Garlic, minced
2 T Smoked Paprika or 1 T Liquid Smoke
1 T Dried Leaf Oregano
1 T Cayenne Pepper
1 T Dried Thyme
3 T Kosher Salt
2 T Ground Black Pepper
1 T Onion Powder
1/4 C Wheat-Free Tamari
2 T Worcestershire Sauce
1 T Onion, finely minced
2 t Chili Powder

If spicy is your "thang," use some red pepper flakes, too

Try a hot marinade for a change. It only requires boiling the marinade and then putting the meat strips in the mixture for a couple of minutes, instead of "marinating" the meat overnight in the cold mixture as you would normally do.

You can use a dehydrator or even your own oven to make the jerky. If you use your oven, plan to use the 150-160 degree setting for 6-8 hours.

Use wire racks to lay out the meat strips with spaces between them, or a broiler pan if you don't have wire racks. Put something under them to catch any drippings. Be sure to turn the strips after about 3 hours or so. When the strips start to look like jerky (darker and harder), turn off the heat and let it cool.

When your jerky is cool, here's where that vacuum sealer can really pay for itself. Jerky will keep in those vacuum-sealed packs in the fridge for at least two months if not three, and even longer in the freezer. If you use zippered plastic storage bags, I'd expect to have it keep for about half as long.

Almond Meal and Flour

Buy raw almonds and an inexpensive burr grinder at Costco and you can make cheap almond flour. You will need to freeze the flour in a zippered baggie to bring out only when you want to use it, get the amount you need for your recipe, and put it right back in the freezer.

Almond Milk

Overnight, soak a cup of almonds in water. The next morning, blanch the almonds in boiling water and remove skins. Place in blender with 4 cups of water or so and pulse until smooth.

Almond Butter

Roast 3 pounds of raw, unsalted almonds on cookie sheets in a 350 degree oven for 10 minutes. Cool for 30 minutes before pulsing on the high setting in a food processor until smooth.

Apple Delight

2 C Unsweetened or Homemade Apple Juice
3 Large Apples
2 Cinnamon Sticks

Preheat oven to 250 degrees. Bring apple juice and cinnamon sticks to a low boil while you slice the apples into 1/8 " thick pieces. Use a slotted spoon to insert the apple pieces into the mixture, cooking them until the apples look almost translucent. Remove apple slices from liquid, dry with paper towels, and lay on wire racks. Set racks on middle shelf and just as with the jerky recipe, place a baking sheet underneath in case of drips. Bake for about 30 minutes until apple slices are almost dry to the touch and appear golden brown. Cool and enjoy!

Coco Crack

1 C Cacao or Cocoa Powder
1 1/2 C Pecans or Macadamia Nuts
1 C Coconut Oil, Melted
1 T Organic Mexican Vanilla
Stevia to Taste

Combine all ingredients together. Spread on a baking sheet lined with parchment or waxed paper and put in the freezer. Break it up into individual pieces when it is hard.

Variations: Add some coconut manna, a couple of tablespoons of Heavy Whipping Cream if you eat dairy, or even some unsweetened coconut flakes.

Non-Dairy Coffee Creamer

Make your own! Use your Magic Bullet (or food processor) for this one. Open a can of coconut milk; add an egg and a couple of tablespoons of coconut oil, and mix. This thick and creamy concoction will keep for a week in the fridge.

Freeze Staples for Later

Did you know that you can freeze garlic? Fill quart-sized freezer containers three-fourths full of peeled garlic, then pour olive oil over the cloves until just covered, Place the garlic straight into the freezer, and it can be defrosted a little at a time. You can also use the oil, which is now infused with garlic, in pesto or other sauces. Don't worry about the more transparent look that the frozen cloves take on; they taste just the same as before freezing.

You can even freeze eggs if you know that you can't use them all in time, before they will go bad. Crack the eggs into a bowl, beat them and pour into ice cube trays to freeze. Pop out the frozen egg cubes and consolidate into zippered freezer bags.

Appendices

These pages contain references that you might want to keep handy by making extra copies of the pages from the book.

Shopping List Staples to Keep on Hand

Copy this page to keep on the refrigerator or in the kitchen, to check or circle something when you finish the last of it. Take to the store.

Ground beef, steaks, roasts, chicken breasts, wild-caught fish and shrimp, eggs, tuna, bacon or other sugar-free pork

Coconut oil, butter, ghee, EVOO, lard

Dairy items (preferably raw) if you eat it: heavy whipping cream, feta cheese, cheddar cheese

Onions, avocados, mushrooms, red peppers, zucchini, lettuce, spinach, asparagus, tomatoes

Berries, lemons, limes, apples

Tomato paste, diced tomatoes, no-sugar salsa, red and green

Minced garlic, kalamata olives, sea salt, coarse black pepper, other spices like cilantro (great detox), basil, chili powder, oregano, and cumin

Coconut flour, almond meal/flour, almonds, almond butter, walnuts, pecans, pine nuts

Coconut milk, chicken broth, bone broth

Organic or Non-Organic Reference Cards

Copy this page and the next and carry it with you to the store to help you remember what really needs to be organic.

Organic Is Best

- **Apples**
- **Celery**
- Cherries
- Grapes (Imported)
- Lettuce
- Nectarines
- Peaches
- Pears
- Spinach
- **Strawberries**
- Bell Peppers

Bold indicates higher need for buying organic due to more pesticides.

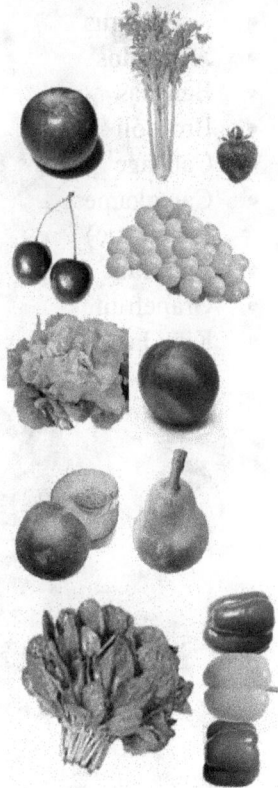

Copy this page and carry it with you to the store to help you remember what can be bought non- organic.

Non-Organic Will Do

- **Asparagus**
- **Avocados**
- Bananas
- Broccoli
- Cabbage
- Cantaloupe (Domestic)
- **Eggplant**
- Grapefruit
- Kiwi Fruit

- **Mangoes**
- Mushrooms
- **Onions**
- Papayas
- **Pineapples**
- Sweet Potatoes
- Watermelon

Bold indicates low levels of pesticides and the least need for buying organic.

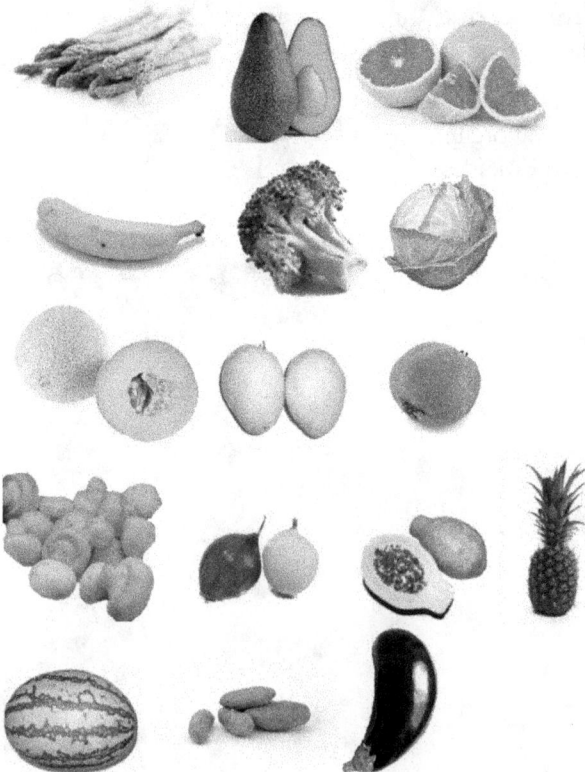

What Spoils Fastest?

These tables are separated by fruits or vegetables.

Fruits

Fruit	Refrigerator	Freezer
Currants	1-2 days	8-12 months
Persimmons	2-3 days	8-12 months
Figs	2-3 days	8-12 months
Berries	2-3 days	8-12 months
Cherries	2-3 days	8-12 months
Pineapples	2-3 days	4-6 months
Cherimoyas	2-5 days RT	8-12 months
Guavas	2-5 days RT	8-12 months
Papayas	2-5 days RT	8-12 months
Bananas	2-5 days RT	8-12 months
Mangoes	2-5 days RT	8-12 months
Plantains	3-5 days RT	8-12 months
Apricots	3-5 days	8-12 months
Avocados	3-5 days	8-12 months
Grapes	3-5 days	8-12 months
Kiwis (Chinese Gooseberry)	3-5 days	4-6 months
Nectarines	3-5 days	8-12 months
Peaches	3-5 days	8-12 months
Pears	3-5 days	8-12 months
Plums	3-5 days	8-12 months
Lychees	1 week	8-12 months
Passion Fruit	1 week	8-12 months
Star Fruit (Carambola)	1 week	8-12 months
Melons	1 week	8-12 months
Pomegranates	2 weeks	8-12 months
Citrus Fruits	2 weeks	4-6 months
Cantaloupe	2 weeks	8-12 months
Apples	1 month	8-12 months

Vegetables

Vegetable	Refrigerator	Freezer
Mushrooms	1 week	8-12 months
Yucca (Cassava)	1-2 days	8-12 months
Turnips	2 weeks	8-12 months
Asparagus	2-3 days	8-12 months
Bok Choy	2-3 days	8-12 months
Cilantro	2-3 days	8-12 months
Kohlrabi (leaves)	2-3 days	8-12 months
Okra	3-5 days	NR
Rhubarb	3-5 days	NR
Purslane	3-5 days	4-6 months
Broccoli	3-5 days	8-12 months
Brussels Sprouts	3-5 days	8-12 months
Greens (Collards, Swiss Chard, Kale, Mustard, Turnip, etc.)	3-5 days	8-12 months
Squash, summer	3-5 days	8-12 months
Zucchini	3-5 days	8-12 months
Cucumber	4-5 days	NR
Yam	1 week RT	8-12 months
Chilies	1 week	NR
Lettuce	1 week	NR
Spinach	1 week	NR
Artichokes	1 week	8-12 months
Cauliflower	1 week	8-12 months
Celery	1 week	8-12 months
Eggplant	1 week	8-12 months
Kohlrabi (stems)	1 week	8-12 months
Leek	1 week	8-12 months
Peppers	1 week	8-12 months
Tomatillos	1 week	8-12 months
Tomatoes	1 week	8-12 months
Onions, green	1-2 weeks	NR
Cabbage	1-2 weeks	NR
Green Beans	2 weeks	NR

Vegetable	Refrigerator	Freezer
Parsley	2 weeks	NR
Radishes	2 weeks	NR
Beets	2 weeks	8-12 months
Carrots	2 weeks	8-12 months
Parsnips	2 weeks	8-12 months
Squash, winter	2 weeks	8-12 months
Jicama	2-3 weeks	8-12 months
Nopales	3 weeks	NR
Sweet Potatoes	3 weeks NR	8-12 months
Onions, yellow, white, red	1-2 months RT	8-12 months
Rutabagas	2 months	8-12 months

RT= Room Temperature

NR = Not Recommended

Refrigerator Drawer Reference to Copy

Drawer 1

Ethylene-Producing

Foods that emit lots of ethylene (the colorless, odorless gaseous hormone that all fruits and veggies give off) include apples, apricots, avocados, unripe bananas, cantaloupe, cherimoya, figs, honeydews, nectarines, papaya, peaches, pears, plums, and tomatoes. Ethylene causes ripening.

Drawer 2

Ethylene-Sensitive

Separate the list above from this list, which are the foods that are extra sensitive to the effects of ethylene. These include ripe bananas, broccoli, Brussels sprouts, cabbage, carrots, cauliflower, cucumbers, eggplant, kiwi, lettuce (and other leafy greens), parsley, peas, peppers, summer squash, sweet potatoes, and watermelon. You don't want these to spoil faster.

That's exactly why you've got two crisper drawers at a minimum in your refrigerator!

Resources

Use these handy links to find these in your area:

- Local farmer's markets http://tinyurl.com/FindaFM

- Local co-ops http://tinyurl.com/FindYourCoop

- Farm shares like CSAs (Community Supported Agriculture programs) http://tinyurl.com/FindaCSA

- Healthy meats from local farmers http://tinyurl.com/EatWild

Also by Harmony Clearwater Grace

HCG Diet Made Simple

Your Step-By-Step Guide Beyond Pounds and Inches 5th Edition

The HCG Diet Book of Secrets

Stabilizing After HCG and Staying Slim Forever

Coming Soon from Harmony Clearwater Grace!

Paleo Pronto

Fast and Fabulous Primal Meals in Minutes

www.ingramcontent.com/pod-product-compliance
Lightning Source LLC
Chambersburg PA
CBHW070351270326
41926CB00017B/4087